Cognitive Therapy for Adolescents in School Settings

The Guilford Practical Intervention in the Schools Series
Kenneth W. Merrell, Series Editor

This series presents the most reader-friendly resources available in key areas of evidence-based practice in school settings. Practitioners will find trustworthy guides on effective behavioral, mental health, and academic interventions, and assessment and measurement approaches. Covering all aspects of planning, implementing, and evaluating high-quality services for students, books in the series are carefully crafted for everyday utility. Features include ready-to-use reproducibles, lay-flat binding to facilitate photocopying, appealing visual elements, and an oversized format.

Recent Volumes

Conducting School-Based Functional Behavioral Assessments,
Second Edition: A Practitioner's Guide
Mark W. Steege and T. Steuart Watson

Evaluating Educational Interventions:
Single-Case Design for Measuring Response to Intervention
T. Chris Riley-Tillman and Matthew K. Burns

Collaborative Home/School Interventions:
Evidence-Based Solutions for Emotional, Behavioral, and Academic Problems
Gretchen Gimpel Peacock and Brent R. Collett

Social and Emotional Learning in the Classroom:
Promoting Mental Health and Academic Success
Kenneth W. Merrell and Barbara A. Gueldner

Executive Skills in Children and Adolescents, Second Edition:
A Practical Guide to Assessment and Intervention
Peg Dawson and Richard Guare

Responding to Problem Behavior in Schools, Second Edition:
The Behavior Education Program
Deanne A. Crone, Leanne S. Hawken, and Robert H. Horner

High-Functioning Autism/Asperger Syndrome in Schools: Asessment and Intervention
Frank J. Sansosti, Kelly A. Powell-Smith, and Richard J. Cowan

School Discipline and Self-Discipline:
A Practical Guide to Promoting Prosocial Student Behavior
George G. Bear

Response to Intervention, Second Edition:
Principles and Strategies for Effective Practice
Rachel Brown-Chidsey and Mark W. Steege

Child and Adolescent Suicidal Behavior:
School-Based Prevention, Assessment, and Intervention
David N. Miller

Cognitive Therapy for Adolescents in School Settings
Torrey A. Creed, Jarrod Reisweber, and Aaron T. Beck

Cognitive Therapy
for Adolescents
in School Settings

TORREY A. CREED
JARROD REISWEBER
AARON T. BECK

THE GUILFORD PRESS
New York   London

© 2011 The Guilford Press
A Division of Guilford Publications, Inc.
72 Spring Street, New York, NY 10012
www.guilford.com

Printed in Canada

This book is printed on acid-free paper.

Last digit is print number: 9   8   7   6   5   4   3   2   1

The authors have checked with sources believed to be reliable in their efforts to provide
information that is complete and generally in accord with the standards of practice that are
accepted at the time of publication. However, in view of the possibility of human error or changes
in behavioral, mental health, or medical sciences, neither the authors, nor the editor and publisher,
nor any other party who has been involved in the preparation or publication of this work warrants
that the information contained herein is in every respect accurate or complete, and they are not
responsible for any errors or omissions or the results obtained from the use of such information.
Readers are encouraged to confirm the information contained in this book with other sources.

Library of Congress Cataloging-in-Publication Data

Creed, Torrey A.
  Cognitive therapy for adolescents in school settings / by Torrey A. Creed, Jarrod Reisweber,
and Aaron T. Beck.
    p. cm.—(The Guilford practical intervention in the schools series)
  Includes bibliographical references and index.
  ISBN 978-1-60918-133-8 (pbk.: alk. paper)
  1. Cognitive therapy for children.   2. School mental health services.   3. Emotional problems
of children—Treatment.   4. Behavior disorders in children—Treatment.   5. Cognitive
Therapy—methods.   6. Education, Special—methods.   I. Reisweber, Jarrod.   II. Beck,
Aaron T.   III. Title.
  LB3430.C74   2011
  371.7′13—dc22
                                                                      2010048042

MIX
Paper from
responsible sources
FSC® C004071

About the Authors

Torrey A. Creed, PhD, is a clinical psychologist with the Psychopathology Research Unit at the University of Pennsylvania and the Center for Family Intervention Science at the Children's Hospital of Philadelphia. She is also Project Director and Lead Trainer in the Child Expansion of the Beck Initiative, a collaboration between the University of Pennsylvania and the City of Philadelphia's Department of Behavioral Health and Mental Retardation Services, which trains community therapists to conduct cognitive therapy for prevention and treatment of a variety of problems and disorders, including suicide, depression, trauma, substance misuse, depression, and anxiety in youth. Dr. Creed's primary research interests include cognitive therapy, treatment outcome with youth and families, suicide, and trauma. She has provided direct intervention for children and adolescents in schools and trained mental health care professionals to practice cognitive therapy in a range of school settings.

Jarrod Reisweber, PsyD, is Acute Services Coordinator for veterans in Philadelphia and a program director in the Psychopathology Research Unit at the University of Pennsylvania. His clinical interests include suicide prevention, substance abuse treatment, intervention programs for externalizing males, and cognitive therapy for individuals with schizophrenia. Dr. Reisweber has trained clinicians to conduct cognitive therapy in school, correctional, and community mental health settings; presented internationally on anger management and suicide prevention programs for high school students; and published on interventions and consultation in high schools.

Aaron T. Beck, MD, is University Professor Emeritus of Psychiatry at the University of Pennsylvania School of Medicine and the founder of cognitive therapy. He has published more than 21 books and over 560 articles in professional and scientific journals. Dr. Beck is the recipient of numerous awards, including the Rhoda and Bernard Sarnat International Prize in Mental Health (2003), the Albert Lasker Clinical Medical Research Award (2006), the Gustav O. Lienhard Award (2006), the American Psychological Association Lifetime Achievement Award (2007), the American Psychiatric Association Distinguished Service Award (2008), and the Robert J. and Claire Pasarow Foundation Award for Research in Neuropsychiatry (2008). He is President of The Beck Institute for Cognitive Therapy and Research and Honorary President of the Academy of Cognitive Therapy.

Acknowledgments

We would like to thank the City of Philadelphia's Department of Behavioral Health and Mental Retardation Services and Community Behavioral Health for their collaboration on the Beck Initiative, a program through which community clinicians are trained to conduct cognitive therapy for prevention and treatment of a variety of problems and disorders. This program and the trainees were the inspiration for the development of this book. Specifically, we would like to thank Drs. Arthur C. Evans, Gail Edelsohn, Marc Forman, and J. Bryce McLaulin as well as Regina Xhezo for their exceptional commitment to bringing evidence-based practices to community mental health. We would also like to thank the clinicians and administrators at the Warren E. Smith satellite clinic located at Frankford High School in Philadelphia, and the clinicians and administrators at Silver Springs–Martin Luther School in Plymouth Meeting, Pennsylvania, for their valuable insights. Finally, we acknowledge Heath Hodge's contributions to the diagrams and handouts in this text, which support our mission of bridging the gap between the research and practice sides of psychology.

Torrey A. Creed: I would like to thank my mentors, Drs. Aaron T. Beck, Guy S. Diamond, and Philip C. Kendall, for their guidance and support in building a professional path that is meaningful, fulfilling, and balanced. I am also grateful—always—for the love and support of my parents, Trevor and Cathryn Weiss. Finally, I thank my son, Jeremy Creed, for his love, advice, and wonderful distractions.

Jarrod Reisweber: I would like to express appreciation to Dr. Aaron T. Beck, an outstanding coauthor, clinical supervisor, and mentor. Above all, I must also thank Erika D. Curiel for her continued support and love; without it, my work on this project would not have been possible.

Aaron T. Beck: I would like to dedicate this work to my wife, children, grandchildren, and great-grandchildren.

Contents

3. Cognitive Techniques   57

4. Behavioral Techniques   99

5. Making Cognitive Therapy Happen in the Schools   122

List of Figures, Tables, and Appendices

FIGURES

TABLES

APPENDICES

Cognitive Therapy for Adolescents in School Settings

CHAPTER 1

An Overview of Cognitive Therapy

For more than 50 years, cognitive therapy (CT) has been studied and refined, resulting in a therapy model that is effective for a wide range of disorders and stressors among students. In addition to the scientific evidence that CT is effective, the therapy is structured around a model that clinicians and adolescents themselves have found to be very usable. These factors have led to growing interest in learning how to share CT with mental health professionals in the schools in a way that leads to good outcomes for students.

Training school and community mental health professionals in CT (or any other empirically supported treatment) is a relatively new focus for the research world. Much of the research to date that tests the effectiveness of treatments has been conducted in research labs under highly controlled conditions. Critics noted that although this research showed that CT and other treatments worked under ideal conditions with carefully chosen clients and small caseloads, there was not enough evidence that the treatments would work in the "real world." Therefore, researchers began to examine ways to share these treatments with clinicians working in community mental health centers, schools, hospitals, and other settings with their typical clients to see if the treatments would translate to these environments.

With the push to bridge the gap between researching and providing mental health services in mind, we created the following text that is driven by research, informed by clinical experience, and designed to provide a usable framework for CT in a school setting. We have incorporated feedback from mental health professionals in schools to try to represent the unique challenges and rewards of working with youth in the day-to-day realities of this setting. We have intentionally focused the text on the clinical use of CT, rather than on the research behind the model. However, for readers who are interested in the research that supports this work, a list of recommended readings has been included at the end of each chapter and at the end of the text.

In writing this text, we hope to reach a wide audience of readers working with adolescents in school settings. Many different kinds of professionals may find themselves in this role, including (but certainly not limited to) school psychologists, school social workers, clinical psychologists, school clinicians, mental health support workers, teachers, and others. We have chosen the word *clinician* to refer broadly and inclusively to anyone who might use the CT skills we describe in this book to work with adolescents in a school setting. Although this word may not be exactly the right fit for the varied roles of all readers, our intention is to include all professionals dedicated to helping adolescents in schools make meaningful changes in their lives.

To present CT in a way that can be particularly useful for clinicians in a school setting, we will:

- Present **vignettes** of four adolescents dealing with the kinds of issues you may see in your school, which will be used to work through examples of the ways in which CT can be applied to adolescents in a school setting.
- Present the general **cognitive model**, followed by a discussion of the **terms** and concepts commonly used in CT.
- Explore how to create a CT **case conceptualization** and how you can use that conceptualization to choose specific interventions for your students.
- Describe specific **CT techniques** (both cognitive and behavioral) that can be applied to issues that are commonly seen in a school setting.
- Discuss the **structure** of CT, with a focus on the ways that CT's structure can be particularly effective with the demands of a school setting.
- Examine the question of **parental involvement** in school-based therapy.
- Consider the unique challenges and rewards of working in a **school setting**.

You may notice that we do not explicitly emphasize other essential skills, such as creating a strong relationship with students, expressing empathy, or building trust. These skills are very important in CT, just as they are in most forms of therapy. Without these vital building blocks in place in therapy, clients are not likely to make meaningful change, regardless of how skillfully the clinician chooses and uses interventions. However, these skills are not unique to CT. If you are an experienced clinician, these are skills you have already developed, and if you are training to be a clinician, these skills will be part of your comprehensive training outside of CT. Therefore, this manual will focus solely on the conceptual understanding and techniques that are related to the cognitive model and the cognitive interventions you will use with students.

CHARACTER INTRODUCTIONS

The stories of the following four adolescents are based on the real-life stories of high school students we have worked with. However, none of these stories are the actual stories of one individual student. Instead, we have constructed stories that illustrate some of the issues we often see in adolescents and that represent some of the common, complicated cases we see in the schools. Please reflect on these cases and on how you would work with these students as you read the following four narratives, as they will be referenced throughout the text.

> **Alfred, Anjanae, David, and Michele represent the diverse problems that adolescents in schools may face. We will follow their treatment throughout this book.**

Alfred

Coach Dillman comes to you about Alfred, a 17-year-old Mexican American student whose serious academic difficulties have put him in jeopardy of being eliminated from the wrestling team and losing eligibility for a college scholarship. You have heard other students say that Alfred has recently been using drugs and alcohol at weekend parties. Coach Dillman knows Alfred very well, having coached him for the past 3 years, and he is able to give you the following information.

Coach Dillman describes Alfred as "a good kid who is hanging out with the wrong crowd." The coach notes that in the past Alfred has frequently acted as a good role model for other students and has had a positive influence on the other wrestlers during practice. Coach Dillman states that, "Alfred is sometimes too aggressive, but he was always able to keep that in check in the past." However, after Alfred had a physical fight with another wrestler 6 weeks ago, Coach Dillman threw him out of wrestling practice. Alfred has yet to contact him or return to practice. When he followed up with Alfred's teachers, Coach Dillman learned that Alfred has also been skipping school since that time, and his grades have been dropping quickly. Alfred is now academically ineligible to participate in athletics because of his poor GPA. The coach notes his disappointment about Alfred, remembering that he has always talked about sports as his "ticket out of the neighborhood" in which he grew up.

During the next week, you hear from other students that Alfred has been seen with members of Dogtown, a gang that claims his block as their territory. You ask the coach about this news, and he responds that he is not surprised. Alfred's father left the home when Alfred was a child, and his mother has a significant substance abuse problem, so the coach believes that there is no one at home to guide Alfred and steer him away from trouble. The coach tells you, "This kid thinks he has just two choices available to deal with the 'hood: sports or gangs."

If you were presented with a student like Alfred, where would you begin? Is there any other information you would want before you met with him? What would you want to do in your first session? What kinds of goals would you have for therapy? And how would you try to move toward those goals? Make a few notes, so that you can refer back as we reference Alfred.

_____

_____

_____

_____

_____

_____

_____

_____

Anjanae

The school nurse calls your office to refer Anjanae, a 14-year-old African American girl in the ninth grade. Anjanae has been in the nurse's office complaining of feeling nausea each morning for the past week, ultimately prompting the nurse to suggest a pregnancy test. The positive result on the test has left Anjanae stunned and upset, which is why the nurse is making the referral.

When Anjanae arrives in your office, she is tearful and tense. After she has had a chance to stop crying and catch her breath, you gather a bit of background information. Anjanae is a high achiever in school, with a 3.7 GPA. However, she describes herself as an average student. She says that her grades are not as good as they should be, because it is a struggle to find time to study or do homework at home. As the oldest of four children, Anjanae is expected to care for her brothers and sisters while her mother works a second shift. She is responsible for making and cleaning up after dinner, supervising everyone's homework, and getting everyone bathed and into bed on time. She is often too tired to do homework or study effectively after finishing with these responsibilities. When she finally goes to bed, she often lays awake for up to 2 hours, worrying about her grades, her family, and safety issues in her relatively violent neighborhood. She also dreads being the center of attention, so if she has a presentation to give in class, she will often be sleepless the night before it is due.

Anjanae has recently become sexually active with a new boyfriend, and she describes this as the only thing in her life right now that she does just for herself. Her pregnancy is a result of this sexual activity. Sitting in your office, she voices fears about her mother's reaction, the impact the pregnancy will have on high school and her college plans, and whether her new boyfriend will continue to be involved with her after he hears the news of the pregnancy.

Which issues would you prioritize in your work with Anjanae? Which issues, if any, do you see as important for her long-term well-being, but not necessary for immediate focus? How would you think about these longer term issues in the context of school-based treatment?

_____

_____

_____

_____

_____

_____

_____

_____

David

Early Thursday morning, you come to your office and see two students waiting at your door. You are greeted by a 14-year-old Caucasian girl, who is sitting next to a 14-year-old African American boy with his head in his hands, hunched over in front of your door. She asks whether they can speak with you, and almost as soon as you walk into your office, she states, "Some of the guys are bullying David and I can't stand it!"

The girl then describes a group of boys who have been targeting David during and after school. "They have been harassing David, and it has really hurt his feelings," she complains. You turn to David and ask why they are harassing him and hear silence . . . until the girl blurts, "They are harassing David because he is different . . . because they are intimidated by the fact that David is gay." You send the girl to class, quickly review David's file, and find out that he has a history of being bullied that dates as far back as kindergarten. David also has a learning disability, which according to previous clinician notes, has affected his self-esteem.

After a few sessions, David slowly begins to trust you and tells you, "I was never good enough and I never fit in." He details the difficulties he has had being African American and gay and how this has resulted in rejection for as long as he can remember. He also describes how difficult it has been for him to find someone who appreciates him for who he is.

In the most recent session, you asked David questions about whether he thinks that he has shut down in school and with friends. He rarely goes out with friends after school, and he sleeps through most of his classes. While this has been an ongoing problem with David since middle school, it has gotten worse recently. David stated, "Basically, I feel totally different from everyone else. I can't learn the same way they do, and the idea of dating is a nightmare. I just want to give up on all of it."

How would you help David? What would you target? How would you take into account the way that culture may be influencing David's situation? What kinds of interventions might be best for David, and how would you choose those interventions?

_____

_____

_____

_____

_____

_____

_____

_____

Michele

Midway through the afternoon, a 16-year-old Caucasian girl enters the clinic, wiping away tears from her face. She asks if she can sit in the clinic for a while because she has been unable to stop crying for the past 20 minutes in class. When you ask her name, she introduces herself as Michele, but she does not make any eye contact with you. You agree to let her sit in the clinic for a few minutes while you finish with another student, and when you return after 15 minutes, you find Michele sitting on a chair in the corner of the clinic, still crying. Concerned, you ask her to come into your office to talk with you.

Michele is very slow to trust you or to talk about herself, but over the course of several meetings with you, she finally reveals that she is deeply depressed. She cries easily and often, has had trouble eating and sleeping, and feels completely exhausted. In her saddest, darkest moments, Michele thinks about killing herself as the only way to escape from the difficult things in her life; when she is feeling really down and frustrated, she sometimes cuts herself with a razor blade on her thighs. These cuts are never deep enough to put her life in any danger, but they bleed and appear to be leaving scars.

Michele tells you that she has two main things that make her feel this sad. First, from ages 8–11, her mother's boyfriend sexually abused her. When Michele told a friend about the abuse, the friend confided in an adult who ultimately reported the abuse to Michele's mother and the police. Michele's mother accused her of trying to steal her boyfriend and still blames her for the relationship coming to an end. Michele's sadness over her difficult relationship with her mother, as well as her confusion about the sexual abuse, are often on her mind when she becomes so sad that she thinks of killing herself.

The second thing that Michele blames for her sadness is that she sees herself as "a fat pig" even though her weight is average for her height. Michele goes through cycles of trying not to eat so that she can lose weight, and then becomes so hungry that she eats large quantities of food at one time. When she has eaten a lot of food, she becomes very upset with herself, telling herself that she will be fat forever because she has no willpower, and that no boy will ever be interested in her. In the short term, this causes her to be so upset that she often cuts herself on her upper thighs. In the longer term, Michele seeks sexual attention from boys to reassure herself that she is attractive. Her attention seeking often ends with her having sex with a boy to reassure herself that he is interested in her. However, when the interest does not last for long after the sex, she becomes upset and determined to starve herself to become more attractive. These cycles of starvation and bingeing, plus casual sex and rejection, often leave her feeling very sad and alone.

Several of Michele's classes are with boys she has had sex with, which leads her to think about all of these issues while she is in class. Once she starts to think about the things that make her sad, she starts to cry and has a hard time stopping, so she has asked if she can come to your office when she feels that way.

How would you respond to Michele's request to sit in your office when she starts to cry in class? How would you help Michele make a change in these cycles she is repeating? Which of the different issues she is dealing with would you start with? How would you prioritize her different concerns? To what degree are you, as her clinician, legally obligated to notify the authorities?

_____

_____

_____

_____

_____

_____

_____

_____

Summary of Vignettes

Alfred, Anjanae, David, and Michele represent just some of the complex situations and concerns that may bring a student into counseling at school. Some of the problems may be best described as disorders, while others are caused by difficult situations at home, at school, or in other areas of their lives. CT has a model flexible enough to be used with any of these students in a way that can guide the interventions you choose and the way therapy progresses. The model will also help you answer the kinds of questions we asked at the end of each vignette. Many of the answers guided by CT may be similar to the answers you would give now, without CT guiding your decisions. Other answers may change when you look at them from a CT perspective. Overall, the cognitive model will offer a framework for therapy that is broad enough to work with the range of difficulties students present, and offers guidance that is specific enough to be effective with the unique needs of the adolescent sitting in your office.

AN INTRODUCTION
TO COGNITIVE THEORY AND THE COGNITIVE MODEL

People are constantly thinking about the world around them and the way they fit into that world, even if they are not often aware that they are doing so. These thoughts, which may be just below the conscious level, have a profound impact on the ways in which we feel and behave. Cognitive clinicians work with students to bring these types of thoughts to the surface, so that students can actively evaluate them. Thoughts that are accurate or helpful are strengthened, while those thoughts that are distorted or unhelpful are modified to be more helpful. Focusing on thoughts and the beliefs that influence those thoughts helps students to think in ways that lead to more desirable behavior and feelings. Figure 1.1 introduces the ways in which thoughts, feelings and behavior in a situation are related to each other in an ongoing cycle. This concept will be reviewed in much greater detail in later sections.

In the general **cognitive model**, an event triggers the beginning of the cycle (Beck, 1964). The event could be virtually anything, including the alarm clock going off in the morning, being asked on a date, or feeling hunger pangs. That event triggers a thought in the student's mind that generally comes unintentionally and automatically. The thought may not even be noticed by the student. Next, there is an emotional response to the thought; then based on the thought and emotion, a behavior occurs. That behavior can, itself, be an event that triggers a thought, followed by an emotion and a behavior, and the cycle continues. Unaware of this process, the student may think that the triggering event caused the emotion ("It made me feel so angry!" or "That made me really nervous,") and that he or she is helpless to change those responses to the situation. Understanding this process can give us a way to make changes in the cycle, so that we can make choices about our reactions. A reproducible version of this model can be found in Appendix 1.1 at the end of the book.

To examine this process in a more concrete way, let's use the cognitive model to understand Michele. Michele enters the cafeteria during her lunch period and passes a table full

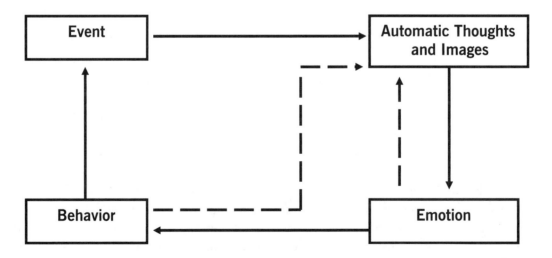

FIGURE 1.1. The general cognitive model.

of boys who all burst into laughter as she walks by. This event (hearing the boys start laughing as she walks by) triggers a number of thoughts in Michele's mind. She says to herself, "I *know* they're laughing at me. They think I look like a big fat pig in these

> ***Situations*** **themselves do not cause us to have certain feelings. It is our *thoughts* about the situation that lead to the feelings.**

jeans—I never should have worn them. Besides, I bet Jay told them that we hooked up. I'm sure they think I'm a total slut, too." Michele may also have images flash through her mind, including a distorted image of her body or an image of herself kissing Jay. Michele may not even realize that these thoughts and images are running through her mind. Often, the first thing we actually notice is a strong emotion. Michele becomes sad and embarrassed as soon she starts thinking about the boys' laughter and what they might be discussing. Based on the thoughts running through her head and her strong negative emotions, Michele buys two lunches and quickly eats both for comfort, sitting alone and feeling sad throughout the meal. Overeating feeds back into this cycle, because it strengthens her beliefs that she has no control over her food intake or her weight. Withdrawing and eating her lunch alone, rather than sitting with her peers, also strengthens her beliefs that no one wants to be with her. These beliefs, combined with her sadness and embarrassment, trigger Michele to seek out a boy for casual sex over the weekend in an effort to reassure herself that someone could be attracted to her. Engaging in casual sex, which is often followed by a lack of respect from the boy, could further strengthen her belief that she is not worthwhile. These strengthened beliefs are likely to cause Michele to continue to withdraw, become more depressed, overeat for comfort, and seek out relationships that are ultimately damaging for her. As illustrated in Figure 1.2, this can create a system that continues to fuel itself, becoming further embedded in Michele's view of the world and herself over time.

Now suppose that on Monday morning, you check in with Michele and she shares the story of the boys laughing in the cafeteria. If you are using CT, Michele might learn to

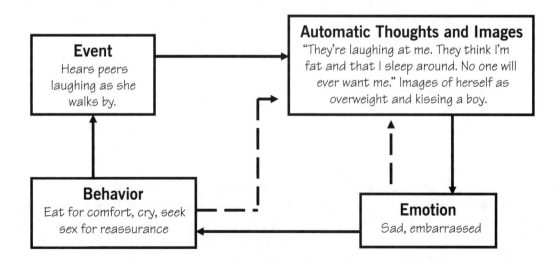

FIGURE 1.2. The general cognitive model: Michele in the lunchroom.

identify these statements she is making to herself, explore and evaluate her beliefs about her relationships with other people and with food, use relaxation or distraction to help calm her emotions when she is upset, and then use coping skills to seek out more healthy interactions with her peers. Regardless of the specific outcome of her attempt to create new healthy relationships, you and Michele would gain new information that would help her to make changes and learn about herself. Successful coping would give her evidence that those negative things she was saying to herself were not completely true, and unsuccessful coping can give both of you more information about where she needs to gain more solid coping skills.

Extending this example for one more step, imagine that Michele has decided to go to a party on Friday. When she arrives at the party, she tries to talk with Alex, a boy whom she finds attractive. However, Alex walks by Michele without acknowledging her. Returning to the general cognitive model, this event (not being acknowledged) triggers a series of thoughts followed by an emotional and behavioral response. However, there is a wide range of thoughts that Michele might have. For example, she may think to herself, "I'm such a fat loser. He doesn't want anything to do with me. I should have just stayed home." These thoughts may lead to feelings of sadness, and Michele is likely to withdraw, socially isolate herself, eat to feel better, have sex for reassurance, or even cut herself. In an alternative scenario, imagine that Michele has worked with you to build her CT skills. Therefore, when the triggering event occurs, Michele says to herself, "He probably just didn't hear me. Besides, if he did hear me and ignored me, that's his issue and his loss. Either way, I'm proud of myself for coming to the party instead of sitting at home, feeling sad and alone." These thoughts may lead to very different feelings than the first scenario, such as a sense of self-respect and a willingness to try to form relationships with people who value her for who she is. In each scenario, the initial event was the same. Michele's way of thinking about the situation made the difference, leading to two very different outcomes. (See Figure 1.3.)

CT uses this cognitive model to understand an individual student's way of thinking about him- or herself, other people, and the world, to understand how those thoughts influence that student's feelings and behaviors, and to identify which of these thoughts are causing difficulties in the student's life. CT then uses a variety of student-tailored strategies to help students modify thoughts so that they reduce the difficulties and increase strengths.

INTRODUCING THE COGNITIVE MODEL TO STUDENTS

One of the unique aspects of CT is that it is very transparent. As cognitive clinicians, we want our students to understand the cognitive model and how it works, and we spend time really explaining and discussing the model with students. Some clinicians find this idea to be strange. After all, the student is not training to be a clinician, right? Wrong! Our goal is to have students ultimately become their own clinicians so that they will be able to explore and evaluate the thoughts and beliefs that could cause them problems down the road. After all, we all have thinking patterns and underlying beliefs that can cause us problems—that's just part of being human. Learning how to work with those thoughts and beliefs so that they no longer get in our way is a skill that can really serve our students for a lifetime.

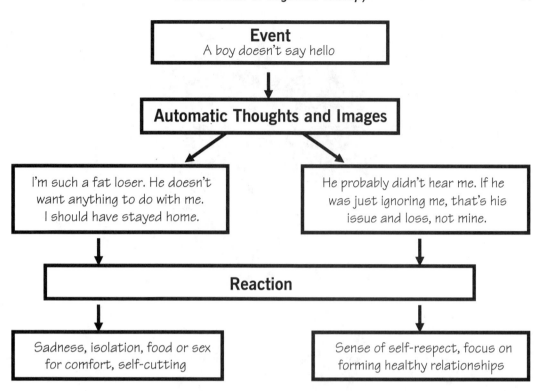

FIGURE 1.3. The general cognitive model: Alternative ways of thinking.

The cognitive model can be explained to students in many ways, but there is a simple story that has resonated particularly well with the many clinicians we have trained and the many students we have worked with. We introduce that story here, but please keep in mind that this story is only one example. You can modify this story to make it more appropriate for any given student. After we present the rollercoaster story, we will discuss how it can be changed to meet yours and your students' needs.

The Rollercoaster Story

"One day last summer, two friends decided to spend the day at an amusement park. After an hour or two of fun, they came to the part of the park where the big rollercoaster was located. Jeremy ran to get in line, and Trevor followed slowly behind him. As they were waiting in line, they looked something like this. . . . "

> The rollercoaster story is one way of helping students understand the connections among situations, our thoughts, and our reactions.

[The clinician can draw a picture to illustrate Jeremy and Trevor, use a picture cut from a magazine, act out the behaviors, etc. One example of an illustration is shown in Figure 1.4. The aim is to show that Jeremy looks happy and excited and Trevor looks scared. The clinician should not *name* the emotion, though, as you will see below.]

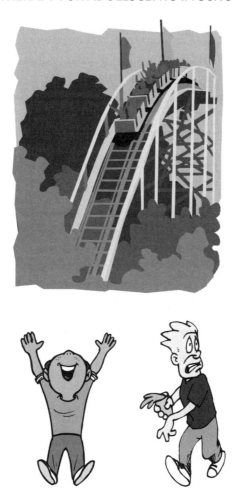

Jeremy   Trevor

FIGURE 1.4. Jeremy and Trevor.

"How do you think Jeremy is feeling?" [Look for the student to say Jeremy is excited, happy etc. Be sure to help the student name *feelings* and not *thoughts*, like "I can't wait!"]

"How do you think Trevor is feeling?" [Look for the student to say Trevor is scared, worried, etc. Again, help the student name feelings instead of thoughts.]

"Excellent job! I think you're right—Jeremy is feeling really good about getting on the rollercoaster, but Trevor looks like he doesn't feel good about it at all. So here's the interesting thing. Lots of students tell me in the beginning of counseling that there are things in their lives that are *making* them feel a certain way—just like the rollercoaster is *making* Jeremy excited and *making* Trevor scared. The thing I wonder is, how can the same rollercoaster be *making* two guys feel two totally opposite ways? It's the same rollercoaster! I wonder if instead of the rollercoaster being in charge of how they feel, it might be something else. Now let's look at something else that's going on with Jeremy and Trevor. What is Jeremy saying to himself while he's standing in line? And what is Trevor saying?"

[Here, we are looking for the (automatic) thoughts that each boy is having when he looks at the rollercoaster. If you have drawn Jeremy and Trevor, you can draw a thought bubble over each of their heads such as we might see in cartoons (see Figure 1.5). If you are telling the story, have the student pretend to be Jeremy and Trevor and guess what's going through each of their minds. The goal is to have the student identify two different sets of thoughts. Jeremy should be thinking about things going well on the rollercoaster, and Trevor should be thinking about things going really badly.]

"I think you're right. Jeremy is probably saying something to himself about how good this ride is going to be, and Trevor probably thinks that something pretty bad is going to happen. He may even have images in his mind of himself throwing up, or the rollercoaster falling right off of the tracks. So I wonder . . . maybe what's happening here is not that the *rollercoaster* is making these guys feel how they feel, but instead, the way they are *thinking* might be doing it. Do you think that's possible?

"So now let's try something else. What could Jeremy say to Trevor to help Trevor feel a little bit better about riding the rollercoaster?"

[Here, we're looking for anything that might help Trevor cope with his worry. Examples include "It'll be OK. I'll sit with you"; "You rode one almost as big last year even though you were scared, and you ended up loving it!"; and "Go prove to yourself that you can do it!" If the student suggests something that would lead to Trevor avoiding the rollercoaster ("You don't have to go. You can wait for me over there."), ask whether that's going to help Trevor face rollercoasters better next time, or if next time, he'll be even more scared. The goal is to have Trevor feel better about the ride.]

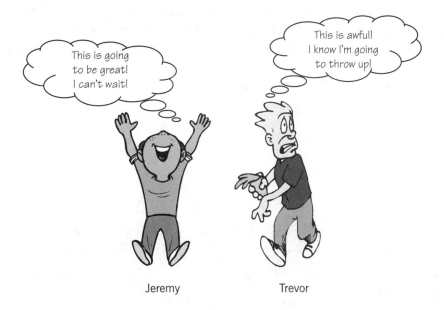

FIGURE 1.5. Jeremy and Trevor with thought bubbles.

"Great! I think that you're right—if Jeremy tells Trevor that he's faced tougher things than this and ended up feeling proud of himself for being brave, Trevor will probably feel a little better about going on the ride. I'm not saying he'll suddenly love rollercoasters, but if he switches from telling himself, 'This is going to be awful. I know I'm gonna throw up!' to 'I can handle this. It's only a 60-second ride,' he's probably going to feel a lot better.

"In the work we'll do together, we will begin by helping you do some of this for yourself. We're going to take a look at the kinds of things you say to yourself in different situations and how those thoughts make you react. Then we'll see if there are other things you can say to yourself—like Jeremy said to Trevor—to help you feel a little better in those situations. Over time, we'll see if there are patterns to the kinds of things you tell yourself, and then work on shifting the ones that aren't working so well for you. How does that sound?"

The example above is just one way that illustrates these ideas for students in a concrete way. You can create an example like this, using anything that two people may feel differently about. Feel free to get creative and use examples that are relevant to something the student enjoys (or really dislikes), something current in the news or pop culture, a type of music or food, or anything else. The important thing is that the student understand the model. A great way to check the student's understanding is to ask him or her to tell you a rollercoaster story using something besides a rollercoaster. For example, a similar story could be told about two adolescents who see a dog sitting on the corner. One may feel scared, and the other may be a dog lover and feel happy about the idea of walking by a dog. See if the student can generate some things that the happy adolescent could say to the scared adolescent to make the situation easier to handle. For older, more mature, or more cognitively sophisticated students, you can also explain the model as it was described here. However, we have found that students respond well to the sense of fun that is part of the rollercoaster story. Use your clinical judgment to find a way of explaining the model that works well for you and your students. On the lines below, try to develop a version of the rollercoaster story that would catch the attention and interest of one of your students, and help them to understand the model.

_____

_____

_____

_____

_____

_____

_____

COGNITIVE THERAPY CONCEPTS

A solid understanding of the main CT concepts will help you to begin planning student-tailored strategies. The most important of these concepts are automatic thoughts, intermediate beliefs, core beliefs, and compensatory strategies (Beck, Rush, Shaw, & Emory, 1979). These terms are interrelated because an understanding of one term builds on the understanding of the others. The concepts can be thought of as similar to an iceberg (Figure 1.6), not unlike the description of psychological structures commonly attributed to Freud. Reactions, including compensatory strategies, behavior, and emotion, are the tip of the iceberg that shows above the water. These reactions can usually be observed without much effort. Automatic thoughts are just below the surface of the ocean, and they can be easily seen if you know where to look in the water. Intermediate beliefs are further down the iceberg, but they can be seen by a person who dives below the surface. Core beliefs are near the bottom of the ocean and are much harder to reach.

Automatic Thoughts and Images

Of the three levels of our thoughts and beliefs, **automatic thoughts** are the easiest to access. Automatic thoughts typically lie just below conscious awareness, although with a little practice, these thoughts can be brought to the conscious level for examination. Automatic thoughts and images are the quick, evaluative thoughts and images that occur in response to outside events (Beck et al., 1979). These automatic thoughts and images may be positive or negative, helpful or unhelpful, accurate or inaccurate. However, there are three common categories into which automatic thoughts often fit (Beck, 1995).

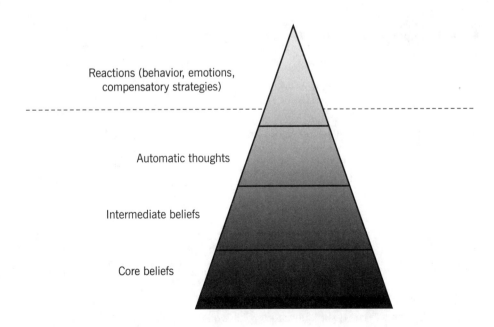

FIGURE 1.6. A representation of the relationship between the main CT concepts.

1. Negative automatic thoughts and images often represent situations in which a person is assuming the worst, often with little or no evidence to support the assumption.
2. Permissive automatic thoughts and images are ideas a student has that allow or excuse behavior that would otherwise cause feelings of guilt or discomfort.
3. Coping thoughts and images help a person to handle difficult situations in a healthy way.

Returning to the examples above, Michele's negative automatic thoughts when she heard the boys laughing at lunch were, "I *know* they're laughing at me. They think I look like a big fat pig in these jeans—I never should have worn them. Besides, I bet Jay told them that we hooked up. I'm sure they think I sleep around, too." She also had a very unflattering image in her mind of herself looking unattractive and overweight. When she later went to the party and a boy did not speak to her, her automatic thoughts could have been negative ("I'm such a fat loser. He doesn't want anything to do with me. I should have stayed home,") or coping ("He probably didn't hear me. If he was just ignoring me, then it's his issue and his loss.") Table 1.1 is a very short representative list of examples of other various automatic thoughts. In reality, automatic thoughts are as varied as people and as the situations in which they find themselves.

These quick reactions and judgments are often followed by a strong emotional, physiological, and/or behavioral reaction. In fact, a good way to help students begin to identify automatic thoughts and images is to have them stop when they have a strong reaction and ask themselves, "What went through my mind just then?" (Beck, 1995). Thought records, which help students to see how their thoughts relate to situations and feelings, are an excel-

TABLE 1.1. Examples of Automatic Thoughts

Negative	Permissive	Coping
"I blew it."	"I've earned it!"	"I will just do my best, and that will be enough."
"He doesn't want me here."	"Just this once . . . "	"I'm proud of myself for trying."
"There's no use trying."	"I held up my end of the bargain—it's not my fault if they didn't."	"No matter what, I can learn from this, and try again if I need to."
"She thinks I'm stupid."	"Everyone else does it, so I may as well."	"Everyone makes mistakes."
"I can't do it."	"They blame me for it, so I may as well do it."	"I may do even better than I expect!"
"I don't fit in here."	"If she doesn't know, it won't hurt her."	"I can handle this."

lent way for students to begin to recognize and track their automatic thoughts (Beck et al., 1979). For clinicians, completing their own thought records is often an interesting and engaging way to understand automatic thoughts and their impact on our responses. Thought records will be discussed in more detail in Chapter 3.

Can you identify automatic thoughts that you sometimes find yourself having? Remember to look at situations where you had a strong emotional reaction, and then ask yourself, "What went through my mind just then?" What was the situation? What did you catch yourself thinking in that moment? If you have a hard time identifying automatic thoughts, don't worry. We will spend much more time looking at automatic thoughts in later chapters.

_____

_____

_____

_____

_____

_____

_____

_____

Cognitive Errors

Although automatic thoughts can be accurate, there are common errors in logical thinking that high school students (and people of every age) often have, leading to automatic thoughts that are not accurate or helpful. These **cognitive errors** occur more frequently in persons who are in emotional distress or have a psychiatric disorder than in people without emotional concerns (Beck, 1976). In working with high school students, these cognitive errors may be referred to as "thinking traps." Thinking traps are common patterns of thinking adolescents may experience that lead to automatic thoughts that are problematic or unhelpful. Table 1.2 presents some of the common thinking traps that adolescents may experience. A reproducible thinking traps worksheet can be found in Appendix 1.2 at the end of the book. At first, the identification of exactly which cognitive errors are occurring is not the primary focus in therapy. Instead, the key is recognizing that there are errors in the logic behind the thoughts, because the errors are a sign that the thoughts could be explored and changed to be more helpful.

TABLE 1.2. Thinking Traps

The repeat	Thinking that if something happened once, it will always happen the same way.
"It's all about me"	Blaming yourself for bad things that happen, even when they actually have nothing to do with you.
The pessimist	Expecting that things will always turn out for the worst.
Selective sight	Not seeing the good parts of a situation, but picking out all of the dangerous or bad things that could/did happen.
Ignoring evidence	Picking out the evidence that tells you that the worst thing is going to happen, instead of looking at all the evidence to decide what will happen.
The jumper	Jumping to conclusions before getting all the facts about a situation.
The mind reader	Reading minds, but not in a good way—such as deciding that someone is thinking something bad about you without any evidence.
Shoulds	"Should" thinking—"I *should* start a fight with every person who crosses me" or "I *shouldn't* ever get mad."
The crystal ball	Predicting what will happen in the future, and that things will probably go wrong.
A perfect disaster	Thinking that if something is less than perfect, it is a complete failure.

Do you recognize any of these thinking traps in your own thinking? Which one(s)?

_____

_____

_____

Which thinking traps do you see most often in your students?

_____

_____

_____

But This Student's Automatic Thought Is True!

As we mentioned above, not all automatic thoughts are wrong or based on thinking traps. Sometimes automatic thoughts can be true, helpful, or both. For example, Alfred may often think to himself, "I'm a talented wrestler. It could be my ticket out of this neighborhood." This thought is a helpful and possibly accurate thought, so as a clinician, we do not need to help him modify it. On the other hand, David may think to himself, "My learning disability means I'll never read as fast as other people, which must mean I'm stupid"; these thoughts may lead to feelings of sadness and frustration. The first part of this thought may be accurate, but thinking it still seems to be getting in his way and leaving him feeling bad, particularly since it leads him to conclude that he is stupid. Clinicians who are first learning CT often have a hard time figuring out what to do when a student has a thought that is true (because challenging it will not be effective or realistic), yet is also getting in the student's way, as for David. In the intervention chapters, we will talk about cognitive and behavioral strategies for helping students deal with thoughts that may be accurate but that are not helpful for them.

Underlying Beliefs

Our automatic thoughts are really expressions of our beliefs about ourselves, others, and the world around us. These **underlying beliefs** can act as a lens through which we see the world, coloring the way we interpret events or expect things to happen (Beck et al., 1979). Underlying beliefs are often

> **Underlying beliefs are the way we understand ourselves, others, and the world around us. Automatic thoughts are quick, evaluative thoughts that are informed by those underlying beliefs.**

formed as a result of an interaction between our genetic makeup and our early life experiences. At this time we are also developing our sense of who we are and how the world works. There are two levels of underlying beliefs: intermediate and core beliefs. However, it can be quite challenging to tease apart intermediate and core beliefs, and in a school setting, you may not have enough time to work with students on such a detailed level. Therefore, intermediate and core beliefs are considered separately here and in the following chapter for clinicians to learn and consider, but in your work with students, you may choose to refer to intermediate and core beliefs together as underlying beliefs.

Intermediate beliefs are midlevel beliefs that lie just underneath automatic thoughts (Beck et al., 1979). When you work with a student to track his or her automatic thoughts, the pattern or common thread that emerges among those automatic thoughts will point to the student's intermediate beliefs. Intermediate beliefs can be thought of as the student's internalized "rules" for how the world works. These rules are often framed as if–then statements, where the student believes that *if* one thing happens, *then* it will lead to a specific result (which may be positive or negative). For example, if we look at Michele's automatic thoughts and actions, we can start to make an educated guess about her intermediate beliefs. She thinks things like, "*If* I have sex with that boy, *then* it will mean that he likes me," and "*If* boys do not like me, *then* I am worthless." Based on those thoughts, we could take a good guess that she believes that (1) her value as a young woman is based on approval from males, and (2) that having sex with them is a good way to get that approval. She may also believe that sex is a sign that she is not as physically unattractive as she fears. As clinicians, we can check these assumptions with our students, gently. Over time, examining automatic thoughts will continue to point toward the intermediate beliefs that our students have. Our first educated guess may not be right, but after we share it with a student, we can work together to examine the possible intermediate belief to see if it corresponds to how the student sees the world. As with automatic thoughts, these intermediate beliefs may be true and helpful, true but not very helpful, or untrue. For thoughts that are untrue or unhelpful, we will use cognitive and behavioral strategies to help students test out these intermediate beliefs and change them to ideas that are more helpful. We will talk about ways to work on those in the intervention chapters.

Core beliefs are the foundation of how we see ourselves, others, and the world (Beck et al., 1979). These rigid and absolute beliefs are usually developed in childhood and based on our experiences. For instance, a child who is repeatedly exposed to developmentally inappropriate tasks that are too difficult may develop the belief that she is incompetent. A child who is repeatedly pushed away in response to efforts for attention may develop the belief that he is unlovable. Some core beliefs may be shaped directly or indirectly by students' families, with effects across many generations. For example, a father's beliefs may shape how he interacts with his wife and children. The children, while watching the marital interactions and how their father behaves with them, will develop their own beliefs. The children's beliefs may be shaped directly ("Never depend on anyone!") or indirectly (watching cycles of violence). Each of the siblings in the family may also develop a distinct set of beliefs that are different from each other and from their parents' beliefs, based on their own unique experiences in and out of the home. In Chapter 2, we discuss the ways in which core beliefs can be identified and understood, and in Chapters 3 and 4, we consider intervention techniques for modifying core beliefs.

Compensatory Strategies

Students develop a set of strategies, or behaviors, that they use to deal with their underlying beliefs and to live according to the "rules" of their world. Examining how students cope with these beliefs can help you and your students understand how some of those thoughts and behaviors developed.

Compensatory strategies generally fit into one of three categories: maintaining strategies, opposing strategies, and avoiding strategies (Beck, 1995). Maintaining strategies support the core belief that they reflect. Opposing strategies are ways of trying to prove that the core belief is wrong. Finally, avoiding strategies are ways in which students try to not activate the core belief at all. Students may use more than one compensatory strategy to manage their core beliefs. For example, take a look at Figure 1.7. This student may deal with the core belief ("I'm a failure.") through any of the three types of compensatory strategies.

For example, Michele's intermediate belief ("If boys do not like me, then I am a worthless person.") and core belief ("I am unlovable.") led to her behavior—promiscuity. Her strategy was to have casual sex with boys to get attention and approval from them. She believed that getting this approval would mean that she was not worthless. In addition, she believed that having boys be physically attracted to her would mean that she was not as unattractive as she feared. Seeking reassurance that she was not worthless or unattractive was related to Michele's core belief that she is completely unlovable and her intermediate beliefs about how she should manage that core belief. Which categories of compensatory strategies was Michele using?

Core Belief

"I am a failure."

Maintaining Strategy

"I overprepare for tasks (like presentations and tests) because I am such a failure, I need to overdo. That way, I never challenge my belief and therefore I continue to believe it."

Opposing Strategy

"I challenge myself to try something new. I am trying to prove that my belief is wrong, which guides my behavior in situations."

Avoiding Strategy

"I avoid any tasks that seem difficult. If I am never challenged, I never have to find out whether it is true that I am a failure."

FIGURE 1.7. Examples of compensatory strategies.

Unfortunately, Michele's strategy had a significant flaw in it. Rather than receiving approval and attention from her behavior, boys often dismissed her after casual sex, and Michele interpreted this response as rejection based on her underlying beliefs about herself. First, she took the rejection as a sign that she is, in fact, worthless and unlovable. Second, she saw the rejection as evidence that she is a physically unattractive "fat pig." These interpretations led to a new set of strategies, which included starving and bingeing to control her weight. These interpretations also led to increased feelings of sadness and hopelessness, and strengthened the intensity of her underlying beliefs about herself.

Understanding how and why these behaviors, or compensatory strategies, developed can help to build a clearer sense of how students understand and deal with their view of the world. New behaviors can be developed to deal with beliefs in a way that does not cause problems for the student or reinforce unhelpful beliefs. In this way, you can choose strategic interventions on the basis of your understanding of each student.

At this stage, some of these ideas may seem really complicated and abstract. (Are you having any automatic thoughts about it?) Don't worry about the details of how each of these pieces come together to make CT work. Instead, look at this overview as an introduction to some of the things you will be learning and practicing throughout the rest of this book. Cognitive counseling may seem complex at first, but by the time you get to the end of this book, you will be familiar with these concepts and have learned ways to flexibly apply them with your students.

LEVELS OF CHANGE
IN COGNITIVE THERAPY IN SCHOOL SETTINGS

As you already know, counseling with students in a school setting is different from traditional outpatient therapy in many ways. The impact of the unique qualities of school counseling are addressed throughout the book and are a focus of Chapter 5. A particularly important quality of school counseling is the level of change that a student or a clinician might expect from counseling sessions. For example, a student like Anjanae may enter counseling to solve her immediate problem (an unplanned pregnancy). She and her clinician may have different ideas about how to prioritize interventions for some of her other, somewhat less immediate concerns (perfectionism, worry, taking a parenting role with her brothers and sisters). Some school counseling centers will vary in their policies or expectations about how long students can be seen for treatment or the kinds of topics that are appropriate for treatment in a school. Students will vary in how open they are to talking about bigger picture issues, how aware they are that change can be made on a larger scale, and how sophisticated their thinking is. Clinicians will also vary in how comfortable they are with deeper levels of change, how much time they can invest in an individual case, and how they see their role as a school clinician.

These differences between counseling centers, clinicians, and students can lead to very different treatment focuses. Counseling for some students may focus more on behavioral, thought, and mood change to resolve the student's current problems. Counseling for other students may move into a deeper level of making major changes in how the student sees him- or herself, others, and the world. Cognitive therapy can be effective for change on both levels, but in the limited amount of time available to most clinicians for treating individual students, it is important to have a clear sense of the target from the initial sessions.

Throughout this book, we will refer to ways in which techniques can be used to target more immediate, current concerns or broader, deeper level change. This is not to imply that both levels of change cannot happen at the same time or that the goals of therapy cannot shift from one level of change to the other. Instead, we are suggesting that you clarify your treatment goals as to the level of change that you and the student are working toward, and that you allow those goals to guide you in choosing and shaping interventions.

Returning to the example of Anjanae, both immediate and longer term concerns could be a focus of treatment. In a very immediate sense, Anjanae has an unplanned pregnancy to manage. She needs to make a number of decisions and then deal with the outcomes of her decisions. She also has issues that are less crisis level but that seem to also be interfering with her current functioning, including concerns about her many responsibilities at home, her academic performance, and her worries about safety, and to name a few. Digging deeper, Anjanae's core beliefs about herself and the world around her are likely to be fueling some of her current concerns. For example, it could be helpful for her to explore her ideas about perfectionism. As a student with a 3.7 GPA, and in the face of her many other responsibilities, what does it mean that she describes herself only as an "average" student? Another area for exploration is the ways in which she makes choices about taking good care of herself. She also described her sexual relationship with her boyfriend as the only positive thing she does for herself, but she has been engaging in unprotected sex with him and is now worried about the impact of a pregnancy on her educational plans and her relationships. She also has been assigned so many responsibilities at home that she is taking care of others at the expense of meeting her own needs. What do these behaviors suggest that Anjanae believes to be true about who she is and what she deserves?

_____

_____

_____

_____

_____

Anjanae, like many students, has many complex levels of issues that could be addressed in therapy. A challenge for you, as her clinician, is choosing where to start, where to aim in the longer term, and what to address along the way. We suggest that there are two main ways to organize your goals in CT to deal with these kinds of complexities. Counseling may be anchored on goals related to changes in thinking and behavior patterns or on deeper seated change of underlying beliefs. We are not suggesting that any counseling should be limited exclusively to one or the other of these goals. Instead, being clear about the student's intentions and your intentions will help to guide you in choosing

> Anchoring counseling on goals related to changing *thinking and behavior patterns*, or deeper seated change of *underlying beliefs*, helps to define a focus for counseling.

interventions, giving you an overall direction in counseling. During the process, however, you will probably be doing work in both thinking / behavior patterns and in the deeper-seated beliefs; the choice of where to anchor the therapy will simply determine where the main focus will be. This choice should be guided by the student's goals and priorities, the time and resources you have available to you for intervention with the student, the student's level of cognitive sophistication, and other important factors. Table 1.3 presents some of these decision points. Please note that the decision on how broadly therapy goals should be defined may depend on the state laws and school district codes affecting specific schools. Therefore, as with any type of counseling, be sure to always operate within the legal and ethical guidelines of your specific setting.

Throughout the text, we periodically suggest different approaches based on whether treatment is anchored to the underlying beliefs or to the thinking and/or behavior patterns that get in the way of the student's goals. These suggestions will help you to tailor your work with each student to focus on goals that fit that student's needs. It is also important to

TABLE 1.3. Decision Points to Anchor Counseling

	Thinking and behavior patterns	Underlying belief patterns
Student's goals	Concrete, behavioral focus	Change in perspective or in patterns
Available time and resources	Limited	Less limited
Student's cognitive development	Younger, concrete thinker, less cognitively sophisticated	Able to think abstractly
Student's motivation	Deal with immediate concerns	Long-term change

remember that counseling should generally not focus on thinking and behavioral change to the point where core beliefs are ignored, or vice versa. Instead, you and the student will clearly define the goals of counseling and focus in that direction, using a wider perspective to inform your work toward change.

In our experience, the majority of school counseling cases focus on the more immediate issues, because students usually arrive in the clinician's office to talk about a current problem or concern that they want to resolve during the session. For example, if Alfred were already working with the school clinician the day he was thrown out of wrestling practice for fighting, he might have come to a session to talk about his anger toward the other wrestler and the coach, or to figure out how to deal with his conflict with them. A student who arrives in the clinician's office to talk about deep-seated beliefs that she is worthless or powerless would be much more unusual in most schools, and in many schools, this topic may be seen as inappropriate for ongoing counseling. A referral to an outpatient therapist may be more appropriate. However, having a clear and detailed understanding of how the cognitive model relates to the student's problems is still a key factor in successful cognitive counseling.

Once you understand how the student's thoughts, feelings, and behavior fit into the cognitive model, you can use the model to create a framework for your work together. When a student arrives at to a session to discuss the problems of the day, this model (or case conceptualization, as discussed in more detail in Chapter 2) will allow you to build continuity between sessions. While using the interventions presented in Chapters 3 and 4 to help the student with problem solving or recognizing and challenging thinking traps, for example, you will also consider the way in which the current problem fits into the case conceptualization. How are the student's patterns of thinking, feeling, and behaving contributing to the current problems? Linking the student's current concerns to this bigger-picture understanding will help you to choose interventions that target the underlying beliefs and to help the student begin to recognize the patterns for him- or herself. In this way, daily concerns are dealt with, but systematic progress is also made. Using the case conceptualization in this way stops sessions from becoming a series of "putting out fires" or dealing with the "crisis of the week."

Consider, for example, how this method might apply to your work with David. Below is a simplified version of a cognitive conceptualization you have developed by the end of Session 3. We will talk about how to build a case conceptualization in Chapter 2, but for now, consider the information below. We have listed the information from David's background that is particularly important to the counseling work and the core and intermediate beliefs that we have identified with David (Figure 1.8). Two situations are then described, in which David had a strong reaction that created a problem or distress for him. Looking

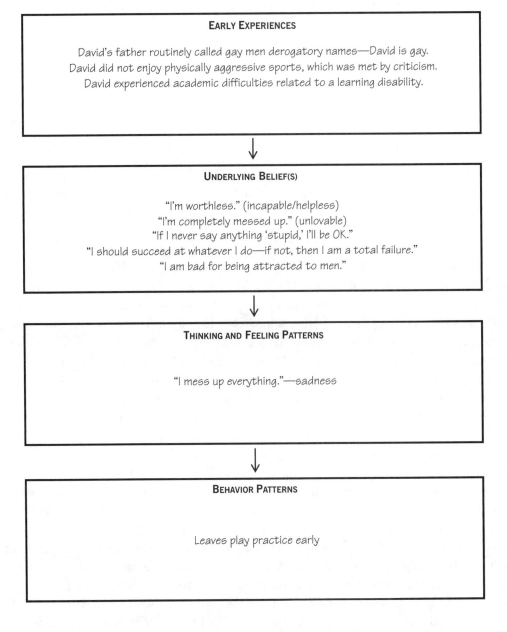

FIGURE 1.8. David's case conceptualization—simplified (based on Beck, 1995).

at distressing situations using the cognitive model can be very helpful for students, as they try to understand their reactions and work toward more helpful ones. For David, two recent distressing situations include a time when David reacted strongly to constructive criticism from a friend about his acting in the school play, and a moment when David found himself attracted to one of his male friends.

When David comes for his fourth session, he tells you about a recent conversation with a friend who gave him feedback during a play practice. David was so upset by hearing the feedback that he left. He is now in trouble with the director, and he is devastated because the play is the one bright spot in his school day. If David came to you with this story, but you were not yet trained in CT, how would you try to work with him during the session?

_____

_____

_____

_____

Some clinicians might listen to David's story and focus on empathizing with him, reflecting back to him that you understand how hard it is to get negative feedback about something you are trying hard to do well. (But would you really understand why it was so hard *for him*, without a cognitive case conceptualization?) Other clinicians might try to think through his reaction to the friend's feedback and understand the friend's intentions. Was the feedback meant to be mean? Helpful? Humiliating? Based on the fact gathering about the friend, those clinicians might help David to decide how to handle the argument. (But how would the two of you really figure out what was going on in this other boy's head?) Still other clinicians would have other approaches to helping David handle this problem. Among all of these clinicians, how would this approach help David when he comes for his next session, still ashamed for feeling attracted to one of his male friends? Without the cognitive model and a case conceptualization, these problems could become a series of disconnected, disjointed problems without any overall progress being made for David.

Now imagine again that David comes for a session and tells you the same story about getting feedback from the friend about play practice. This time, however, you think about David from a cognitive counseling point of view. You think about what you already know about David, his history, and his beliefs about himself and the world. You listen with empathy to his story, and then you both start to explore his reaction to his friend. Instead of trying to guess what his friend really meant by the comments, or having David continue to guess, you ask David whether his friend's comments fit in with David's own beliefs that he usually messes things up, and that once he has made a mistake, he has failed. This kind of exploration will help you both to understand David's reactions to the specific situation and also help him to see how the patterns in his life are linked to beliefs that may or may not be true or helpful. In this way, David can use the counseling sessions to sort out his daily stresses and also learn more about himself on a level that will help him to make lasting change.

In the following chapters, we talk about how to explore these issues with students so that you can have this kind of broad-based understanding. We then look at ways to choose and use interventions for students that will help them to make changes on both immediate and deeper levels.

A BRIEF INTRODUCTION TO THE STRUCTURE OF COGNITIVE THERAPY

One of the unique features of CT is the structure therapists follow from session to session. Chapter 5 details the way in which the structure guides each session, but we present an introduction to the structure here. Without the knowledge in Chapters 1–4, many therapists struggle to make sense of the reason for structuring a session or the components of that structure. Therefore, we first discuss more about the cognitive model and the interventions that follow from a cognitive case conceptualization. Once those building blocks are in place, we describe the session structure as a format for covering all of the important session material in the relatively short sessions (30 minutes or so) that usually take place in a school.

In brief, you may think of the session structure as the skeleton of the session. From session to session, different content provides the details. However, during each meeting, the following will take place:

- Presession Quick Sheet—a worksheet completed by students before session
- Check-in ⎫
- Agenda ⎬ about 5 minutes
- Discussion of agenda items— about 20 minutes
- Homework assignment ⎫
- Summary and feedback ⎬ about 5 minutes

An explanation of each of these components will be provided later. For now, the most important information to take from this list is that CT sessions have a format that is consistent from meeting to meeting. The format creates a routine that will help you and your students to make the best use of your time, creating the greatest possible progress and gains.

SUPPORTING EVIDENCE

Here, and at the end of each of the following chapters, we will review the empirical support for the concepts and techniques that have been presented. In this first chapter, we have presented CT and its underlying model as an effective way of treating a very wide range of problems and disorders. CT and cognitive-behavioral therapy (CBT) are some of the most widely researched psychological therapies, and it would be far beyond the scope of this book to present all of the research that supports the effectiveness of this work. Three of the best sources for reviewing the details of this research are:

- Beck, A. T. (2005). The current state of cognitive therapy: A 40-year retrospective. *Archives of General Psychiatry,62,* 953–959.
- Butler, A. C., Chapman, J. E., Forman, E. M., & Beck, A. T. (2006). The empirical status of cognitive-behavioral therapy: A review of meta-analyses. *Clinical Psychology Review, 26*(1), 17–31.
- Chambless, D. L., & Ollendick, T. H. (2001). Empirically supported psychological interventions: Controversies and evidence. *Annual Review of Psychology, 52,* 685–716.

To summarize some of the specific research findings related to CT and CBT, research has shown that CBT is effective for children and adolescents with problems ranging from anxiety and depression to oppositional behavior. Table 1.4 lists of some of the research that supports the use of CT or CBT for these issues; however, hundreds of research articles

TABLE 1.4. Research Support for CT and CBT

Disorder	Supporting research
Depression (among adolescents and depressive symptoms among children)	Butler, Chapman, Forman, & Beck (2006); Chambless & Ollendick (2001); Grossman & Hughes (1992); Reinecke, Ryan, & DuBois (1998)
Anxiety disorders	Butler, Chapman, Forman, & Beck (2006); Chambless & Ollendick (2001); Grossman & Hughes (1992); Kendall, Hudson, Gosch, Flannery-Schroeder, & Suveg (2008)
Separation anxiety disorder	Chambless & Ollendick (2001); Kendall, Hudson, Gosch, Flannery-Schroeder, & Suveg (2008)
Avoidant disorder	Chambless & Ollendick (2001)
Overanxious disorder	Chambless & Ollendick (2001)
Obsessive–compulsive disorder	March (1995); O'Kearney, Anstey, & von Sanden (2006)
Phobias	Chambless & Ollendick (2001)
Posttraumatic stress disorder	Cohen, Deblinger, Mannarino, & Steer (2004); Deblinger, Stauffer, & Steer (2001)
Attention-deficit/hyperactivity disorder	Barkley (2000); Braswell & Bloomquist (1991)
Conduct disorder/oppositional defiant disorder	Chambless & Ollendick (2001)
Physical complaints not explained by a medical condition (somatoform disorders)	Butler, Chapman, Forman, & Beck (2006); Grossman & Hughes (1992); Moss, McGrady, Davies, & Wickramasekera (2003)

exist for readers who are interested in learning more about the research support for these interventions. Many of the techniques and concepts in this book were developed by cognitive clinicians and researchers over the past several decades and are commonly used by clinicians in outpatient settings, schools, inpatient settings, and other mental health care settings. Please refer to the Supporting Evidence sections in the following chapters and the References (pages 163–168) for a complete list of the sources for many of the cognitive techniques and concepts detailed in this book.

SUMMARY

The cognitive model is the backbone of how cognitive clinicians think about and understand students' concerns and the ways in which change can be made. In this model, thoughts, feelings, and behavior are all connected to each other, and an event or situation can start a chain reaction in the relationships among them. Cognitive clinicians put their primary focus on working with students on modifying their thoughts, feelings, and behavior. There are three levels of thinking, ranging from automatic thoughts that are just below the surface of consciousness, to underlying beliefs (intermediate and core beliefs) that are at the heart of how the student sees him- or herself and the world. The student uses compensatory strategies to manage these underlying beliefs about how the world works. A cognitive clinician focuses on the different levels of thinking to understand why students think, feel, and act as they do and to help students make positive change. Counseling goals are then defined with a shorter term, concrete focus or a longer term, wider focus. The counseling work may still address both short-term and long-term goals, but choosing a focus will help the clinician and students to accomplish the goals of counseling. The structure of a CT session makes it easier to meet those goals efficiently in the time available for counseling.

READER ACTIVITY: THE COGNITIVE MODEL

Understanding the cognitive model is key for both you and the students you counsel. Try to think of a story similar to the rollercoaster story that would demonstrate the idea behind the cognitive model in a way that would engage a student. The story could be removed from the kinds of situations students will bring in to the office (like the rollercoaster or the dog stories), or it could represent something more realistic (like two students being bumped in the hall—one gets angry and one shrugs it off).

_____

_____

_____

_____

_____

_____

_____

_____

_____

_____

_____

_____

_____

_____

_____

_____

How can you use the idea behind the cognitive model to help students think differently about the situations they face every day? Is it realistic to work toward helping students to feel great about every situation, or is it more realistic to help them feel a little better about some of them (like Trevor being able to ride the rollercoaster, but not necessarily love it)? What kinds of situations might students face where feeling a little better about it might be the best goal?

_____

_____

_____

_____

_____

_____

_____

_____

_____

CHAPTER 2

Cognitive Therapy
Case Conceptualization

PSYCHOLOGICALLY SPEAKING,
WHY DO STUDENTS DO WHAT THEY DO?

So far, we have suggested that the environment or situation itself does not cause students to feel as they do. Instead, it is the way that students see or think about their situation that leads to particular emotions and behavior. To illustrate this point, let's look at some of the automatic thoughts that students might have as they enter your office. The following are the thoughts of three different students, of which the student may or may not be conscious.

> Student 1: "Counseling may be helpful, but it may be a waste of time. I'll give it a couple of sessions before I make a decision."

> Student 2: "Meeting with a counselor is a waste of time. She won't get what I'm going through and I'm missing art class."

> Student 3: "I really need some help. The counselor really helped Amy, so maybe she can help me."

Given what you have read so far, you probably can guess that these students would each be feeling differently. What would you guess that each is feeling?

Student 1: _____

Student 2: _____

Student 3: _____

You may have guessed that Student 1 was feeling cautious, Student 2 was feeling annoyed, and Student 3 was feeling interested and excited—based on what they were thinking. As we described in the last chapter, the way people think is directly related to the way they feel. And . . . the way we automatically think about something is directly related to our intermediate and core beliefs. Our intermediate and core beliefs therefore guide much of how we feel, and these underlying beliefs and subsequent automatic thoughts and compensatory behaviors can be diagrammed and understood through what a cognitive clinician calls a **cognitive conceptualization** (Beck, 1995). The cognitive conceptualization usually changes over time as clinicians learn more about their students, as the students learn more about themselves, and as students make changes during counseling. The conceptualization represents a clinician's best current understanding of:

- The student's experiences that results in or are related to the formation of the student's beliefs.
- What a student believes about him- or herself, others, and the world.
- The rules students have to live by, given their core beliefs.
- The thinking patterns, based on deeper beliefs that the student may have at a conscious level or just below a conscious level.

> **Clinicians use a cognitive case conceptualization to diagram a student's background information, underlying beliefs, automatic thoughts, and compensatory strategies.**

In thinking about the cognitive conceptualization, do you find yourself feeling anxious or guarded, wondering "That sounds like a lot of work! Why do I need it?" If you are aware of thoughts like this, we hope that you approach this self talk with an open mind and a thought like, "Hmmm . . . Apparently, the cognitive conceptualization—whatever it is—is part of this approach that has been proven effective, so I'll give it a shot." You may find that a thought like this shifts any feelings of frustration to feelings of curiosity or optimism. If you are not having success with shifting your thinking just yet, hang in there. The following chapters will strengthen your skills for doing so, for students and for yourself!

Before you read on, take a moment to first consider how you currently make sense of the students you work with. Do you try to gain a sense of who they are, why they think and act as they do, and what contributed to their being that way? If you do, you are already conceptualizing in a fashion similar to that of a CT clinician—*great*! Much of what is presented in this chapter may be similar to what you are already doing. If this way of thinking about your students is really different from how you usually approach counseling, we invite you to think about what may be different about this kind of conceptualization and how you could integrate CT or the cognitive conceptualization itself into your work with students.

With the student's cognitive conceptualization in mind, the cognitive clinician will be able to target the behaviors, thinking patterns, or underlying beliefs that are interfering with the student reaching his or her goals. In doing so, cognitive counseling goes beyond what traditional supportive therapy accomplishes, as clinicians anchor their work with students to specific thinking patterns or beliefs that are causing problems in the students' lives.

We use the term **anchor** to convey the fact that counseling overall, as well as each session you have with a student, will be tied to the theme or aspect of the student that you and the student are attempting to change.

For some students, you will anchor the treatment to helping students understand and eventually change the role that *unhelpful thoughts and behaviors* play in their functioning. However, when students are interested in and capable of addressing underlying beliefs, there can be even longer lasting changes when you help them change not only the unhelpful thoughts and behaviors, but also the underlying beliefs that are their foundation. When this occurs, you are anchoring each session to the *underlying beliefs* that are related to their current problems and keeping the students from reaching their goals. The cognitive conceptualization of the student will guide you in choosing how to anchor treatment and which interventions to use. Cognitive counseling that is anchored to behaviors, thoughts, and/or underlying beliefs creates continuity between sessions, and the clinician and student alike will have a clearer view of the targets they are working to change. The cognitive conceptualization that informs this process is described in this chapter, and treatment planning that is anchored to behaviors, thinking patterns, and/or underlying beliefs is described in greater detail in Chapters 3 and 5. A depiction of CT sessions as anchored to behaviors, thinking patterns, and/or underlying beliefs is shown in Figure 2.1.

COGNITIVE CONCEPTUALIZATION

Whether you anchor your sessions to the student's thoughts and behaviors or to the students' deeper underlying beliefs, you will always want to have a preliminary cognitive conceptualization of the student formed by about the third session. Contrary to counseling in a traditional outpatient setting, we have found that cognitive school clinicians may not have enough time to work on underlying beliefs with the majority of students. Even if you are not anchoring your sessions to underlying beliefs, it will still be important to understand how

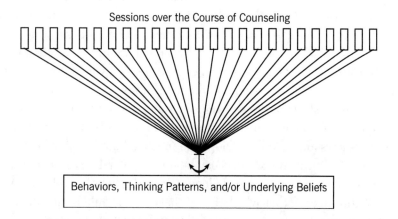

FIGURE 2.1. CT sessions across time.

students' thinking or behavior patterns influence and are influenced by their beliefs. This will help you choose interventions, understand when interventions are not working, and understand why students behave as they do.

Cognitive conceptualizations of the students described in our introductory vignettes are presented throughout this chapter. In fact, you already started working with cognitive conceptualizations and beliefs with David in Chapter 1. Three levels of beliefs are described in detail in the following pages: core beliefs, intermediate beliefs, and automatic thoughts. Core beliefs and intermediate beliefs are students' underlying beliefs about the world and themselves as well as their beliefs about what they need to do to get by in the world. In the following pages, we will first describe core and intermediate beliefs separately, then show how they can be considered together as simply underlying beliefs. Next, we describe how automatic thoughts flow out of these underlying beliefs.

CORE BELIEFS

Core beliefs are the foundational beliefs that a child develops early in life. These beliefs set the stage for later beliefs and thoughts. Core beliefs can be hard to change and are directly related to each student's early childhood experiences. These beliefs about one's self can generally be funneled into one of two categories—beliefs about helplessness or unlovability (Beck, Wright, Newman, & Liese, 1993). For instance, a child who is repeatedly exposed to developmentally inappropriate tasks that are too difficult for her to deal with may develop the belief that she is helpless or incompetent. A child who is repeatedly pushed away in response to efforts for attention may develop the belief that he is unlovable. Alternatively, a child who has experiences of being successful and competent at many of the things she tries may develop a belief that she is capable of navigating the demands of her environment. A child who is accepted and loved is likely to develop the belief that he is lovable.

Many core beliefs may be shaped directly or indirectly by students' families, with effects that span across many generations. For example, consider a little girl who was raised in an abusive home. The violence that followed from anger in that home may have led that little girl to believe that anger is dangerous. She then exhibits a behavioral coping pattern of withdrawing from people expressing anger as a result of automatic thoughts like, "I am in danger!" when she sees her father's anger. Over time, as a way of protecting herself, she withdraws from anyone or any situation in which anger appears. When that child grows up and becomes a mother, she withdraws from her son when he becomes angry, even when that anger is appropriate and not dangerous. Her son observes his mother withdrawing from him whenever he shows anger, and develops the intermediate belief "If I show anger, then people won't love me." In this way, beliefs can be unintentionally passed across generations, taking different forms as they are passed along. When the beliefs of other family members are also added to this mix (a father who believes that anger should be shown as part of discipline, an aunt who reacts to anger with greater anger, etc.), belief systems can become very complicated and very deeply embedded in our personalities.

Other beliefs that originate in childhood are not necessarily passed from one generation to another and are the result of experiences in the child's early life. Let's take a look at Michele for example, who had thoughts like, "No boy will ever truly care about me." As we try to build a cognitive conceptualization of Michele based on her history and the information we learned from her in early sessions, we may hypothesize that those thoughts come from a core belief that she is unlovable and relate to an intermediate belief that sex is the only thing she has to offer others. These beliefs were the result of sexual abuse experiences that were perpetrated by a nonfamily member in childhood, rather than necessarily being a belief system that was passed on from previous generations. Of course, her family may also have beliefs related to sexuality and abuse, but her experience of being abused may have been the biggest factor in Michele developing these beliefs.

Just like automatic thoughts and intermediate beliefs, core beliefs can be (1) true and helpful, (2) true but not very helpful, or (3) untrue. A long-term goal in therapy is to build up and strengthen helpful core beliefs, and to reduce or modify unhelpful ones. Because core beliefs are so deeply ingrained in students (as they are in any other person), and because they are so rigidly and absolutely believed, modifying core beliefs can be a long process. We explore ways to work on changing core beliefs in Chapters 3 and 4 on interventions. Through this discussion, are you beginning to see how early experiences relate to core beliefs which, in turn, affect the way students think about and interact with the world around them?

INTERMEDIATE BELIEFS

Intermediate beliefs are the (usually unexpressed) rules, as a student perceives them, for how the world functions (Beck et al., 1979). As a clinician, you may find it helpful to think of core beliefs as students' "truths" about the world and themselves and intermediate beliefs as the "rules" that they believe exist as a way to deal with their "truths." Those rules then guide the students as they try to navigate the events around them.

Intermediate beliefs are midlevel beliefs that lie just underneath automatic thoughts. When you attempt to help a student become aware of his or her automatic thoughts, the pattern or common thread that emerges among those automatic thoughts will point to the student's intermediate beliefs. Intermediate beliefs can be thought of as the student's internalized "rules" for how the world works. These rules are often framed as if–then statements, where the student believes that *if* one thing happens, *then* it will lead to a specific result (which may be positive or negative).

In the introduction to these concepts in Chapter 1, we looked at Michele's automatic thoughts and actions and started to make an educated guess about her intermediate beliefs. She thinks things like, "*If* I have sex with that boy, *then* it will mean that he likes me," and "*If* boys do not like me, *then* I am worthless." Based on those thoughts, we could take a good guess that she may believe that (1) her value as a young woman is based on approval from males, (2) having sex with males is a good way to get approval, and (3) having sex is a sign that she is not physically unattractive.

COMPENSATORY STRATEGIES

Based on the underlying beliefs that students have about others, the world, and themselves, they develop a set of compensatory strategies, or behaviors, that they use to deal with their underlying beliefs and then live according to the "rules" of their world. These compensatory strategies (Beck, 1995) are behaviors that are sometimes baffling to observe and may be very frustrating to deal with because they seem to work against logic. A key point to remember is that just because these behaviors may go against *your* logic (based on your own set of beliefs) does not mean that there is not logic behind the behavior. Often, when we are able to stop and understand how the world looks when seen through the student's eyes, the behaviors will make sense according to the student's underlying beliefs.

As we mentioned in Chapter 1, compensatory strategies usually fall into one of three categories: (1) maintaining strategies (support a core belief), (2) opposing strategies (ways of trying to prove that a core belief is wrong), and (3) avoiding strategies (ways in which the student tries to keep from triggering the core belief). Students may use more than one compensatory strategy to manage their core beliefs. For example, we looked at one of Michele's compensatory strategies in Chapter 1, as summarized in Figure 2.2.

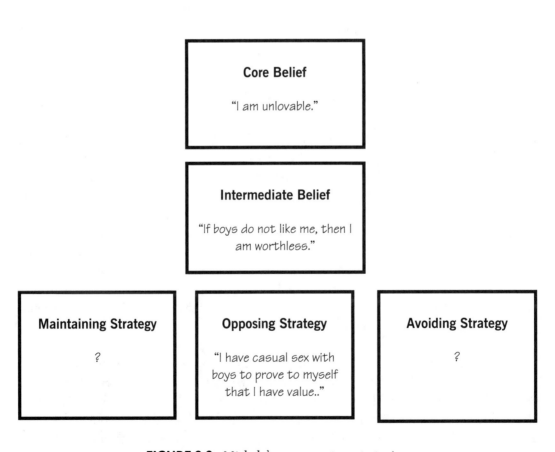

FIGURE 2.2. Michele's compensatory strategies.

Michele's opposing strategy had a significant flaw in it. When boys dismissed her after casual sex, she saw the rejection as a evidence that she is worthless, unlovable, and unattractive. Ultimately, her underlying beliefs about herself were being strengthened. What kind of maintaining and avoiding strategies might you see in Michele? How would these strategies, or behaviors, be likely to affect her beliefs?

Maintaining strategy: _____

_____

_____

How the maintaining strategy affects beliefs: _____

_____

_____

_____

Avoiding strategy: _____

_____

_____

How the avoiding strategy affects beliefs: _____

_____

_____

_____

As her clinician, you would help her watch for these and other behaviors that might seem to be at odds with what Michele really wants. Understanding how and why she uses these strategies, based on her underlying beliefs, can help to build a clearer sense of how Michele understands the world and why she acts as she does. Over time, cognitive counseling can focus on new strategies and interventions to deal with beliefs in a way that does not cause problems for the student or reinforce unhelpful beliefs.

> **A case conceptualization is an evolving picture of the student, representing your understanding of the student at a given point in counseling.**

Take a moment now to look at Figure 2.3. This case conceptualization worksheet (based on Beck, 1995) lists the questions you will want to consider when identifying core and intermediate beliefs, so that you can start to understand your students. We strongly encourage you to use a case conceptualization diagram like this one (included in a reproducible Appendix 2.1 at the end of the book) for each student on your caseload. Case conceptu-

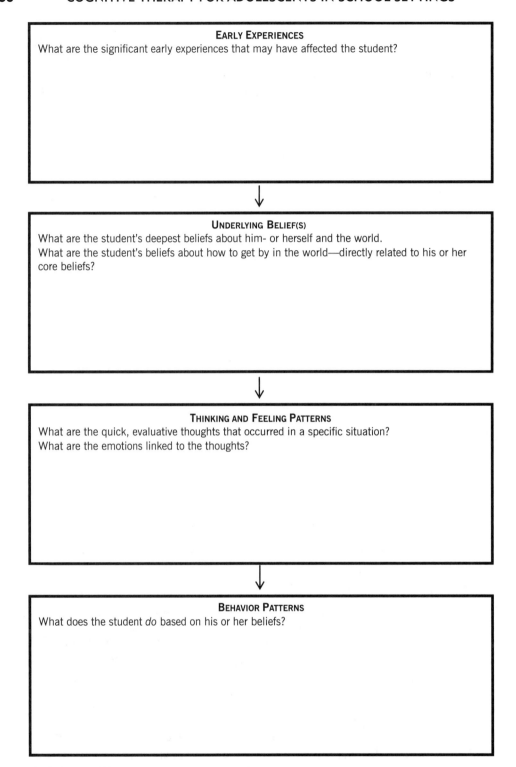

EARLY EXPERIENCES
What are the significant early experiences that may have affected the student?

↓

UNDERLYING BELIEF(S)
What are the student's deepest beliefs about him- or herself and the world.
What are the student's beliefs about how to get by in the world—directly related to his or her core beliefs?

↓

THINKING AND FEELING PATTERNS
What are the quick, evaluative thoughts that occurred in a specific situation?
What are the emotions linked to the thoughts?

↓

BEHAVIOR PATTERNS
What does the student *do* based on his or her beliefs?

FIGURE 2.3. Michele's blank cognitive conceptualization (based on Beck, 1995).

alizations are expected to change over time, as you and the student learn more about the student's thoughts and beliefs and as those thoughts and beliefs change in counseling. After reviewing Michele's story in Chapter 1, think about how you would answer the questions in the blank cognitive conceptualization form (Figure 2.3). After you have filled in your preliminary cognitive conceptualization of Michele, look at our completed cognitive conceptualization (Figure 2.4) to check whether you are thinking along the same lines as we did about Michele.

SIMPLIFYING THE COGNITIVE CONCEPTUALIZATION

Our experience in high schools suggests that most clinicians will not have time to help all students understand the effect of their underlying beliefs. However, when treatment is anchored to changing underlying beliefs, attempting to explain the difference between

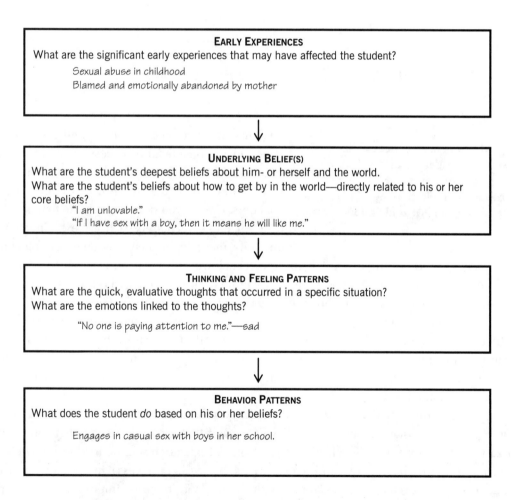

FIGURE 2.4. Michele's completed cognitive conceptualization.

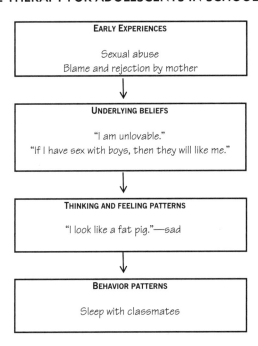

FIGURE 2.5. Cognitive conceptualization presented to Michele.

> **Sharing the case conceptualization with the student is an important way to check in about the student's understanding of his or her own thoughts and beliefs.**

students' intermediate and core beliefs to them is not always beneficial or necessary. As an effective cognitive clinician, it will be important for you to understand the difference between these concepts, even if you do not choose to explain the difference to students. As such, we explained core and intermediate beliefs separately so that you can understand their unique explanatory power. However, we encourage you to combine and describe them as underlying beliefs as you talk with students who are attempting to change these beliefs and to anchor their treatment to such change. The diagram in Figure 2.5 is a condensed cognitive conceptualization that we would share with Michele. Although having a more detailed cognitive conceptualization would still be important for treatment planning, the simplified diagram would be used to communicate the early experiences and underlying beliefs that are interfering with Michele meeting her goals in an easy-to-understand way.

In diagramming beliefs, we recommend that you have a full conceptualization written out prior to the session to mentally guide you as you fill in the underlying belief conceptualization with the student. The full cognitive conceptualization will be held in the back of your mind for guiding sessions and interventions, but will not necessarily be shown to the student. After you complete the diagram with the student, it will be important to compare what you have in your notes to what you and the student agree on. This will help you see where you may need to make changes to your initial cognitive conceptualization hypothesis, and in some cases, also perceive what the students are struggling to see in themselves.

USING YOUR COGNITIVE CONCEPTUALIZATION

Your initial cognitive conceptualization of a student should be developed during the first three sessions with the student, and it should be viewed as a working hypothesis. This hypothesis or educated guess is continually questioned by the clinician in light of what the student brings to each session, and it is changed as the clinician and student learn more about how the student views the world and him- or herself. Over the course of therapy the cognitive conceptualization is also continually refined in light of changes that the student makes in his or her thinking patterns and underlying beliefs (Beck, 1995).

It is unlikely that changes will be made in a student's underlying beliefs in early sessions, before changes in behaviors and thinking patterns are continually demonstrated by the student. As such, most beginning sessions and counseling with high school students in general will focus on changing the thoughts and behaviors of the student. However, this does not mean that focusing on and changing thoughts and behaviors does not affect underlying beliefs. In fact, when your sessions are anchored to underlying belief change, this change will frequently occur as a result of the challenge to the thoughts and behaviors that are interwoven with underlying beliefs. The difference between counseling that is anchored to underlying beliefs rather than to behaviors and thinking patterns is that the student and clinician explicitly review the cognitive conceptualization and how changes in underlying beliefs affect the student. Regardless of what counseling is anchored to, as you and the student work together to find more accurate and helpful thoughts and behaviors, and as the student learns the skill of continuing to use these helpful thoughts and behaviors for themselves, an overall shift in core beliefs will occur.

Let's apply what we know so far to David, another student introduced in our vignettes. David grew up in a Southern Baptist household where gender-typical behaviors were valued and success in school and sports was used as a measuring stick for him and his brothers. David has had academic difficulties for as long as he can remember and was recently diagnosed with a learning disability. Contrary to his family norms, David refrained from participating in sports. David is also gay, which conflicts with his family's values. Now in high school, David has been attending classes less and less frequently. From other students you hear that David thinks that "everyone hates him," and that he believes that he does not fit in with his peers.

Before you read on, take a moment to reread the vignette of David and think about how you would initially make sense of him and how you would approach counseling. In doing this, try and incorporate as much of what you learned from the pages you already read. When you are finished describing how you would make sense of him and how you would approach counseling, take a shot at completing a preliminary cognitive conceptualization (see Figure 2.6).

EARLY EXPERIENCES
What are the significant early experiences that may have affected the student?

↓

UNDERLYING BELIEF(S)
What are the student's deepest beliefs about him- or herself and the world.
What are the student's beliefs about how to get by in the world—directly related to his or her core beliefs?

↓

THINKING AND FEELING PATTERNS
What are the quick, evaluative thoughts that occurred in a specific situation?
What are the emotions linked to the thoughts?

↓

BEHAVIOR PATTERNS
What does the student *do* based on his or her beliefs?

FIGURE 2.6. David's blank cognitive conceptualization (based on Beck, 1995).

How would you initially make sense of David and why he is having difficulties?

_____

_____

_____

_____

_____

_____

_____

What information would you take into account when trying to understand David?

_____

_____

_____

_____

_____

_____

_____

_____

_____

How would you help David address his psychological issues?

_____

_____

_____

_____

_____

_____

_____

_____

_____

What do you think might or might not work for David in counseling?

_____

_____

_____

_____

_____

After reading the following pages, take a look at your approach and preliminary cognitive conceptualization and consider the differences between your approach and conceptualization and ours. After meeting with David a couple of times, reading his file, and collecting background information from other school staff, we had a strong hypothesis about the underlying beliefs that David has about himself and how these beliefs are influencing him. David is probably not aware of his underlying beliefs, but his automatic thoughts will be fairly accessible upon talking to him in counseling. Some of the evidence for our hypotheses came when we saw a well-meaning fellow student provide David with constructive feedback in class. In this and other situations, we noticed that David interpreted constructive feedback as a negative, attack on himself.

Let's look at Figure 2.7, which considers core and intermediate beliefs separately. (A blank cognitive conceptualization form [based on J. S. Beck, 1995] is included in Appendix 2.1 at the end on the book for you to copy and use for formulating your conceptualization of students. Figure 2.7 presents the case conceptualization that we developed after Session 7. An earlier version of this diagram was presented in Chapter 1 (Figure 1.8), but as you will see, we have refined the case conceptualization as we have learned more about David. We conceptualized David as having core beliefs, such as "I am an idiot," which result from not being able to excel in the areas that his father associated with competency. Did you conceptualize something similar? Finally, we included the intermediate belief that "If I'm attracted to boys, then I'm messed up," which David acquired as a result of growing up in an environment with a father who stated that men who are attracted to men are "messed up." We are hoping that you included similar information in the early experiences and intermediate belief sections of your cognitive conceptualization.

The case conceptualization in Figure 2.7 was based on the information gathered by the clinician from conversations with David, information gleaned from other staff members in the school, and case notes acquired from his previous clinician. Some of the information in the case conceptualization may accurately describe David's true thoughts and beliefs, but it is likely that the clinician completing the form also made some mistakes. After all, clinicians are not mind readers, so clinical judgment was used to make the informed guesses (working hypotheses) that led to his developing cognitive conceptualization.

As David and his clinician work together over time, the clinician may discover new factors that should be included in the conceptualization or fine-tune components that are already there. These changes are an expected part of working with a student and, over time, the conceptualization should evolve as a better and better representation of the clinician's

---

EARLY EXPERIENCES

What are the significant early experiences that may have affected the student?

David's father regularly called gay men derogatory names—David is gay.
David did not enjoy physically aggressive sports, which was met by criticism.
Success in school and sports was valued and was the measuring stick for self-worth.
David experienced academic difficulties related to a learning disability.

UNDERLYING BELIEF(S)

What are the student's deepest beliefs about him- or herself and the world.
What are the student's beliefs about how to get by in the world—directly related to his or her core beliefs?

"I'm worthless." (unlovable)
"I'm an idiot." (incapable/helpless)
"I'm completely messed up." (unlovable)

"If I never say anything 'stupid' then I'll be OK."
"I should succeed at whatever I do—if not, then I'm a total failure."
"If I'm attracted to boys, then I'm messed up."
"If I can get everyone to like me, then I'll be good."

THINKING AND FEELING PATTERNS

What are the quick, evaluative thoughts that occurred in a specific situation?
What are the emotions linked to the thoughts?

"I mess up everything." (sadness)
"I'm a freak." (sadness)

BEHAVIOR PATTERNS

What does the student *do* based on his or her beliefs?

Withdraws from peers.
Gives up on classes.
Avoids boys he is attracted to.
Tries very hard to please others.

FIGURE 2.7. David's completed cognitive conceptualization.

understanding of the student. If sessions are anchored to underlying beliefs, David and his clinician could refer back to their modified cognitive conceptualization as a framework for understanding David's reactions to new and ongoing situations.

AUTOMATIC THOUGHTS: SHEDDING LIGHT ON UNDERLYING BELIEFS

As noted in Chapter 1, automatic thoughts are thoughts that lie in the stream of conscious processing. Although most of this chapter described the underlying beliefs from which the automatic thoughts flow, challenging and modifying automatic thoughts will be the primary focus of your work with most high school students. To understand how automatic thoughts relate to core and intermediate beliefs, see Figure 2.8.

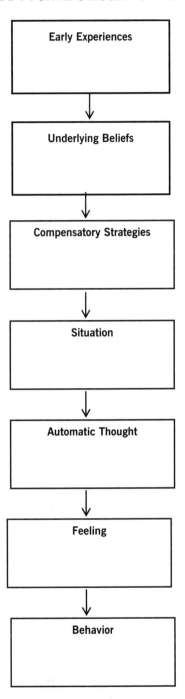

FIGURE 2.8. Cognitive conceptualization affecting automatic thoughts.

Figure 2.8 shows how underlying beliefs influence the way that students think about their situations. With students whose sessions are anchored to changing underling beliefs, the diagram can be helpful in showing them how their thoughts relate to their underlying beliefs, guiding them through examples from their lives. The following narrative presents a clinician attempting to explain to David how his underlying beliefs may relate to his problems, and it takes place in the 10th counseling session. Please note that in a real counseling session, it is unlikely that the conversation would move this quickly or that the student would give such "ideal" answers. However, in the interest of showing how a clinician and student can work together to understand how beliefs play out in a student's life, we present the following simplified narrative. In a real session, your goal would be for the student to reach the same kinds of conclusions, but the process may be slower.

CLINICIAN: David, we have been meeting for a few weeks now, and I'm noticing some patterns. Yesterday, when your friend Jimmy said that you seemed "off" during play practice, you felt pretty bad and left practice early.

DAVID: Yeah, I felt horrible. I said to myself, "I completely mess up everything I do."

CLINICIAN: I get the sense you were really hurt, and I like that you were able to identify the thought that went with that feeling—"I mess up everything I do." I'm noticing a pattern where you get down on yourself pretty quickly. You have even left school a couple times after doing poorly on schoolwork. After we talked about those times you've remembered having thoughts like "I'm an idiot," or "It's no use trying," go through your head.

DAVID: I know . . . this happens to me all the time.

CLINICIAN: Yeah, you get down on yourself and focus in on one comment or grade and forget the fact that you are doing well in many of your classes and have a lead role in the upcoming play. It must be really hard to have those negative thoughts so often.

DAVID: I don't know why I do that—but sometimes it feels like those other good things don't matter.

CLINICIAN: Let's look at your patterns together and see if we can come up with something. Let me explain how I am beginning to understand you, and then you tell me if you think I am getting it or I'm missing it, OK?

DAVID: OK.

CLINICIAN: I would appreciate that. Growing up, your family, especially your dad, seemed to approve of you only when you were doing well in school or being a "guy's guy."

DAVID: Yeah, but I didn't always do well in school and I'm not a guy's guy . . . it seems like I'm always trying for that and falling short.

CLINICIAN: I'm sure that has been really hard to have your skills and abilities not line up with what your dad valued.

DAVID: Yeah.

CLINICIAN: It seems like you were led to believe that the only way to be worthwhile or effective was to be a great athlete or student.

DAVID: Yeah, but I was an actor and a so-so student, and I always felt like I was messed up or an idiot.

CLINICIAN: I think those statements may be some of those underlying beliefs that get triggered when you are at your lower points.

DAVID: Yeah.

CLINICIAN: I have also noticed that you have some beliefs like "Everyone should like me," and "I should be good at everything I do."

DAVID: Yep, my friends keep telling me that it's OK that everyone won't like me—no one is liked by everybody—and Mr. Kuse keeps telling me that every practice can't be a perfect practice. I think they just feel bad for me, though.

CLINICIAN: So, let's take a look at this diagram. It has boxes for us to list the experiences and underlying beliefs that relate to one another and the resulting thoughts you have when you feel bad. (*Shows Figure 2.9 to David.*)

The clinician would then collaboratively diagram out early experiences and underlying beliefs and show how they result in automatic thoughts as indicated in the previous conceptualization. This cognitive conceptualization was created collaboratively, with the clinician drawing as much information from David as possible, while helping David to figure out its placement in the different sections of the diagram. While doing so, the clinician would

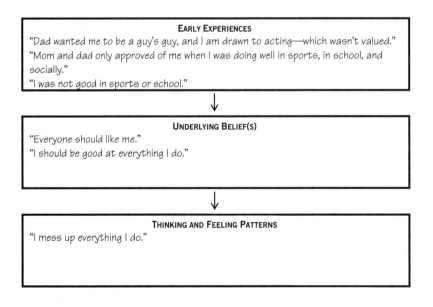

FIGURE 2.9. Counseling with David.

continually check with David to see if what they are writing makes sense to him, and if any of it may be wrong.

CLINICIAN: Now that we have this drawn out, is there anything that we should add to or take out of the diagram? I want to make sure that I am not getting anything wrong or putting words into your mouth.

DAVID: No, this actually makes sense.

CLINICIAN: So can you see how, when someone says you had a bad practice or expresses something negative, that you make meaning out of it in a way that brings you back to negative beliefs about yourself?

DAVID: Yeah, it's not always me, sometimes it's just the way I am making sense of it . . . making sense of it in a negative way.

Once again, anything David does not agree with should be explored, so that the evolving conceptualization feels like a fit for him. This helps to ensure that the diagram is correct and that it is understood by the student. When working with students like David who have their treatment anchored to underlying beliefs in addition to thoughts and behaviors, this diagram should be referenced and updated when problems arise in future sessions so that the diagram becomes more accurate and nuanced and students become more aware of why they react as they do.

When working with students who do not have their treatment plan anchored to their underlying beliefs, you will still fill out a full cognitive conceptualization, but this cognitive conceptualization will not necessarily be presented to these students. Instead, it will be used to help you think about why students are or are not making progress toward their goals and what interventions and approach you should use in counseling. If you were doing this with David, you would still create a cognitive conceptualization of him, and this would help you understand why he is engaging in some of the thinking traps introduced in Chapter 1 as well as why he finds it difficult to change particular thinking patterns. The direction of treatment and the interventions you choose will be guided by your conceptualization, so that you can change the patterns that are getting in the way of his meeting his goals.

COGNITIVE CONCEPTUALIZATION, TREATMENT ANCHORS, AND THE PRESESSION QUICK SHEET

You may not have the time to focus on changing underlying beliefs with many of your students. Counseling sessions in a high school are usually shorter than the traditional weekly 50 minute hour in outpatient settings, and high school students frequently come to the clinician's office immediately after they experience a problem that they are hoping the clinician can address. This context sets the stage for counseling that is anchored to patterns and/or underlying beliefs while simultaneously allowing the clinician to address the immediate concerns of the student.

In our experience, students often come to the clinician's office because of an immediate problem they are having, like fighting with their parents, academic difficulties, conflict with peers, and so on. These problems are frequently seen by the student to have end-of-the-world consequences. Students seek help to make these problems go away, and while this may be one of your immediate goals, you can facilitate longer lasting positive change by helping students see how their current problems relate to their behavior patterns, thinking patterns, and in some cases, underlying beliefs. For instance, when a student routinely shows up at your door with academic difficulties caused by a tendency to avoid stressful or challenging situations, you may focus on thoughts or avoidance behaviors, while simultaneously addressing the immediate concern. This method addresses the immediate issue while also helping the student understand the "what and why" that underlies the pattern of problems.

With some students who are less invested in therapy, younger, or lower functioning, you may want to focus only on their thinking and behavior patterns, but with higher functioning students you may be able to address their behavior, thinking patterns, and underlying beliefs. This approach will help you move from "putting out fires" to modeling how students can understand and address difficulties so that they are equipped to "put out their own fires" in the future. While this method may slow down the problem-solving process initially for the clinician and student, it decreases the demand on counseling in the long term. This understanding, coupled with being taught cognitive strategies, will eventually help students internalize the understanding that they have the tools to address their difficulties with limited or no need for clinician support. Strategies for identifying and changing thinking patterns and underlying beliefs are described in Chapter 3 and strategies for changing behavior patterns are presented in Chapter 4.

To help students understand the thinking and behavior patterns that are related to their problems and serve as the "anchor" for their treatment plan, we recommend asking students to fill out a Presession Quick Sheet (see Figure 2.10). The Quick Sheet, which will

The Presession Quick Sheet helps students to reflect on thought, feeling, and behavior patterns and on acquired skills.

be discussed further in Chapter 5, can be completed quickly in the moments after a student arrives to see you. This worksheet requires the student to stop and reflect on the behaviors, feelings, and thinking patterns that relate to the current situation as well as to apply techniques learned in previous sessions. Having students think through the Quick Sheet questions before the sessions reinforces both their ability to apply already learned CT concepts and the active role they can play in addressing their problems. In an effort to begin understanding the Quick Sheet and how it can help students take an active role in addressing the problems (treatment anchors) that are interfering with their meeting their goals, take a moment to reference the one that Alfred created and its relationship to the work that he and his clinician are doing together. (See Figure 2.10.) This Quick Sheet was created by Alfred prior to Session 9, when Alfred presents with a recurring problem of fighting with peers. A reproducible Presession Quick Sheet can be found in Appendix 2.2 at the end of the book.

In working with Alfred for a few months, the clinician noted that Alfred continually writes on his Quick Sheet automatic thoughts like "I've gotta take this guy out." After

Today I want to talk about: Keith tried to come at me in the hallway today.	I am feeling:	Intensity of feeling:
	Happy	Highest
	Angry	10
		9
	Sad	⑧
		7
	Worried	
What I'm thinking about it is: I gotta take Keith out if he thinks he can do this to me.	Excited	6
	Embarrassed	5
		4
	Guilty	3
	Relaxed	2
	Other	1
		Lowest

My best way to deal with it is:
Not sure. I want to take him out, but I know you're gonna say that I should just ignore it or something.

Things I'm thinking about from our last meeting are:
Automatic thoughts—I don't think I have those.

I did _X_ did not _____ do my practice task.

FIGURE 2.10. Alfred's Presession Quick Sheet.

exploring this thought with Alfred, the clinician believes that this is actually related to an intermediate belief that can act as a treatment anchor. The clinician has a strong hunch/hypothesis that Alfred has both an underlying belief that the world is dangerous and an intermediate belief that the only way for him to stay safe is to attack before he is attacked. Alfred's beliefs were true in many situations and helpful when he was younger and growing up in a dangerous neighborhood. Alfred's beliefs resulted in an aggressive behavior pattern that was reinforced by successes in street fights, in wrestling, and when protecting his brothers and sisters. However, his blanket view of the world as dangerous and aggressive response pattern is no longer working for him, nor is it particularly true when he is in school and around people who want to help him. Please keep in mind the Presession Quick Sheet in Figure 2.10 and how this plays an important role in the counseling presented in the following narrative.

CLINICIAN: Great work on your Quick Sheet, Alfred.

ALFRED: Thanks.

CLINICIAN: I noticed that you had another problem this week where you thought that people were trying to attack you before you really found out what was going on. It seems like that's happening a lot?

ALFRED: I guess. I don't exactly want to wait around to find out if someone's trying to fight me. It's better to just show them I can't be pushed around.

CLINICIAN: Yeah, I understand that thinking when I consider what has happened to you. In fact, I think that it relates to an underlying belief that relates to a lot of your difficulties.

ALFRED: Yeah, it gets me into a lot of trouble, but it's true.

CLINICIAN: Thank you for your honesty, and let's take a look at that statement. Have I ever tried to fight you?

ALFRED: No. I usually don't fight with teachers. It's the kids here that give me a hard time.

CLINICIAN: OK. How many kids at this school have you had a fight with?

ALFRED: Maybe 12.

CLINICIAN: Well, there are about 1,400 kids in this school. Twelve is a lot, but out of the whole school, that's less than 1% of the kids.

ALFRED: Fine. I guess it isn't everybody—just some people.

CLINICIAN: Exactly, but it seems like because of the experiences you had with people growing up, you assume that most people who you don't know will try to come after you and fight you. Does that make sense?

ALFRED: Yeah, but how do I tell which ones want to come at me? How do I know which ones aren't coming after me because they know I'm gonna fight back, and which ones I can ignore?

CLINICIAN: Great questions, and we can figure that out, but first I want to make sure that you understand why you do it. In doing so, we will be anchoring our sessions to understanding why you do it, which will lead to you being better at knowing who is coming at you and who you can trust. What results is your becoming your own clinician.

ALFRED: That would be cool—I like the sound of Dr. Alfred, and I hope Dr. Alfred will get back on the wrestling team and out of detention.

CLINICIAN: Sounds like great goals, Doc!

In the next session, the clinician and Alfred would write out on a cognitive conceptualization diagram the early experiences in Alfred's life that contributed to his seeing people the way he does. In doing so, the clinician should describe how it is natural for Alfred to be hypervigilant and aggressive and how this behavior was protective for him because of where and how he grew up. The clinician should be careful to not discredit or challenge the fact that this behavior may still be protective in dangerous situations outside of school. After Alfred demonstrates that he understands how his underlying beliefs were influenced by his childhood, the clinician can help Alfred see how those beliefs are sometimes problematic with techniques like guided discovery (see Chapter 3).

As in any work with adolescents, it is particularly important to use examples that students can understand and/or identify with, and that give them an image to reference as they attempt to change their behaviors, thoughts, and underlying beliefs. Given Alfred's involvement in sports, the clinician may want to use sports figures who are very aggressive when playing or coaching sports, yet calm and collected when at meetings or talking to the press. The clinician will then explicitly review with Alfred how sessions will be anchored to underlying beliefs in addition to the thoughts and behaviors that they were previously targeting. After developing a cognitive conceptualization of Alfred with him, the clinician will also encourage Alfred to think about the role that his underlying beliefs play in daily problems on future Presession Quick Sheets prior to each session.

SUPPORTING EVIDENCE

Case conceptualization is, in essence, the way in which a CT clinician thinks about a student and chooses specific interventions for specific recurring concerns. The use and development of the case conceptualization is based on CT, and research to test the utility of this way of thinking would be very difficult to do. To determine whether case conceptualization is, itself, an empirically supported technique, researchers would compare cognitive therapy, done with or without a case conceptualization, to measure whether the presence of the case conceptualization made a difference in the outcomes of therapy. However, CT without a case conceptualization would not be CT! Instead, the overall therapy is empirically supported (as we described in Chapter 1).

If you would like to read more about the details of case conceptualization and the ways in which is guides a CT clinician's therapeutic choices, we recommend:

- Beck, J. S. (1995). *Cognitive therapy: Basics and beyond*. New York: Guilford Press. This text, written by the director of the Beck Institute for Cognitive Therapy and Research, is an excellent resource for a strong foundational understanding of case conceptualization and is written in a way that readers generally find easy to apply to their cases.

SUMMARY AND FURTHER THOUGHTS

This chapter presented a lot of information about how clinicians can make sense of the students with whom they are working. It began with a brief introduction to the cognitive model that places an emphasis on the thoughts that relate to what students do and how they feel. These thoughts are influenced by the underlying beliefs of the student, which are diagrammed with a cognitive conceptualization. Having a cognitive conceptualization of the students underlying beliefs allows the clinician to understand why students do what they do. When a student's treatment is anchored to underlying beliefs, the student, too, will see the role underlying beliefs play in the way they think, behave, and feel.

The cognitive conceptualization was divided into core beliefs, intermediate beliefs, and automatic thoughts, which will help you map out and understand your students. However, because of the complexity of this method, we suggest that you condense intermediate and core beliefs into underlying beliefs when discussing cognitive conceptualizations with students. With lower functioning students, younger students, or students who are reluctant to delve into themselves, or when faced with time constraints, you may want to anchor your sessions to the thinking and behavior patterns that are explained by your cognitive conceptualization. Counseling that is initially anchored to addressing thoughts and behaviors can be anchored to underlying beliefs in later sessions if it is clinically indicated, and the student and clinician will establish a cognitive conceptualization at that time. Regardless of whether you are anchoring counseling to underlying beliefs, the cognitive conceptualization will serve as an important framework for understanding and empathizing with each student, choosing the most effective techniques, and understanding why students are or are not making progress in counseling.

READER ACTIVITY: COGNITIVE CONCEPTUALIZATION

In thinking about the concepts in the first two chapters of this book, consider which aspects of the cognitive model are consistent or inconsistent with how you made sense of your students prior to reading this book. We also invite you to conceptualize yourself with a cognitive conceptualization. You can use Figure 2.11, Appendix 2.1, or your own sheet of paper. After you complete a cognitive conceptualization of yourself, we ask that you complete the following questions. Try not to read the questions until after you have completed your cognitive conceptualization.

What automatic thoughts and emotions occurred within you as you completed your cognitive conceptualization?

_____

_____

_____

_____

_____

_____

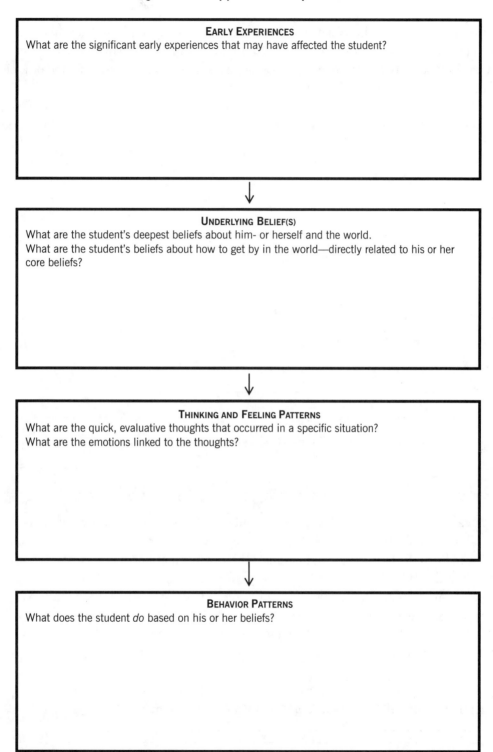

FIGURE 2.11. Clinician's cognitive conceptualization.

We frequently find that this can be a difficult task for clinicians and students alike and hope that completing your cognitive conceptualization will help you empathize with the process that you will be taking your students through and the shame, anger, sadness, and other feelings, that can coincide with this self-reflective act.

What surprised you about yourself when you completed your cognitive conceptualization?

_____

_____

_____

_____

_____

_____

How may your understanding of yourself and your early experiences impact your counseling?

_____

_____

_____

_____

_____

_____

We have found that clinicians' experiences influence the way they conceptualize their students. For example, beginning CT clinicians may have an unconscious tendency to conceptualize their students in a way that parallels their own experiences and conceptualization. If you find that this is the case or if many of your students have similar conceptualizations, review them again and make sure that you are not making hypotheses that are based on your own experiences or automatic thoughts. Instead, you will want to make sure that your student conceptualizations are a reflection of what each unique student brings to sessions—the data that spurs your hypotheses.

If you were to enter your own counseling, how would having this cognitive conceptualization influence counseling, and would it be useful?

_____

_____

_____

_____

CHAPTER 3

Cognitive Techniques

This chapter introduces the cognitive techniques that we have found most effective and useful while working in the school system. It has been our experience that these techniques lend themselves to the unique characteristics of high school students and to the schools themselves. When you are finished reading this chapter, you should have a basic understanding of collaborative problem solving, thought records, thought bubbles, guided discovery, the Three C's, coping cards, and the reverse role play. The last technique presented in this chapter is the downward arrow, and it can be used by clinicians to expose the underlying beliefs that are the psychological foundation and reason for some students' problems.

A DECISION POINT: PROBLEM SOLVING OR INTERVENTION?

Before choosing an intervention to try with a student, one main question must be answered. Is the issue on the table a result of an inaccurate or unhelpful thought or underlying belief, or is the issue a problem situation where the student is having a reasonable reaction (thoughts, feelings, behavior)? When the student's thought or belief is contributing to the problem, cognitive and behavioral strategies will help the student to make changes toward more accurate and helpful thoughts or beliefs. However, one of the most common questions we are asked by clinicians is, what do I do when the student is right? What happens when the issue is a real problem situation in the student's life, instead of something for which changing their thinking can help? When these situations arise, you and the student will move directly into collaborative problem solving.

> When a student's distress is a reasonable reaction to a situation, rather than related to unhelpful or inaccurate thoughts and beliefs, we move to collaborative problem solving.

COLLABORATIVE PROBLEM SOLVING

Collaborative problem solving is a process in which the clinician asks questions in a manner that helps the student identify the problem, determine how to best respond to it, and in some cases, how to change the situation (Beck, 1995). Frequently, collaborative problem solving with a student can be an effective intervention in and of itself. This is especially evident when students' feelings are an appropriate fit for their situation, and it would therefore be counterproductive to try to change the realistic and adaptive thoughts they have in relation to it. For instance, it would be insulting to suggest that students who have suffered the loss of a parent or failed a needed class should not feel grief or sadness—that they should just modify how they think about the situation and somehow feel fine.

No amount of working with thoughts will change the fact that Anjanae is facing an unplanned pregnancy. Trying to talk David through testing his beliefs will not change the fact that he has a learning disability that may make some classes more difficult for him. Instead, students with feelings that match their situations can be helped with problem solving. In doing this collaboratively with your students, you are not only moving toward a solution, but also teaching students how to problem solve, which is a skill that they can apply to future situations. We suggest that it may be best to encourage students to engage in problem solving when the following occur:

1. When the student's emotions are appropriate to the situation.
2. When the student is in a situation that places him or her at significant risk of harm.
3. When you and the student have checked the student's thought and it appears both accurate and useful.
4. When the student is functioning at a lower level and initially finds it difficult to understand how the beliefs, thoughts, and behaviors relate to the problem.

When teaching students to problem-solve, we have found the **ITCH method** (Muñoz, Ippen, Rao, Le, & Dwyer, 2000) to be very effective. This method places an emphasis on establishing different options and then weighing the pros and cons of each method. While doing so may be common sense for many adults, we have found that it is not always common sense for the adolescent in a stressful situation. Therefore, presenting the ITCH mnemonic is a simple method of teaching these skills to adolescents in a way that they may remember and find useful. Figure 3.1 lists the steps that you can use in session. Figure 3.2 is an example of a sheet that students could use during or outside of the session.

As students become more skilled in working through these steps, problem solving will become a more natural process. Over time, the student will not need to move step by step in such a structured way because the process will become more automatic and internalized. When a student experiences difficulties in problem solving, help the student identify the thinking patterns and underlying beliefs that are making it difficult. This will inform your cognitive conceptualization, and you will then need to decide if it will be more fruitful to address problematic thinking patterns and/or underlying beliefs or to offer more direct

ITCHing to Solve a Problem?

- **Identify the Problem:** Collaboratively help the student identify what is happening and what is difficult about the problem.
- **Think about Possible Solutions:** Collaboratively help the student identify some different options he or she can use to handle this situation. Try not to pick only helpful solutions but brainstorm several possibilities.
- **Choose a Solution to Try:** Collaboratively help the student look at the list of possibilities and identify which one makes the most sense. What could get in the way of the student when he or she tries out the solution? What are ways to get over these obstacles?
- **How Well Does It Work?** Prior to trying out the solution, help the student consider in the end what may make the approach successful or unsuccessful. After the student tries the solution, assess the results, and restart the process if necessary.

FIGURE 3.1. The ITCH problem-solving method for use in session (based on Muñoz, Ippen, Rao, Le, & Dwyler, 2000).

Identify the Problem: What is happening and what is difficult about it?

____

____

____

Think about Possible Solutions: What are some different options you can use to handle this situation? Try not to pick only helpful solutions but brainstorm several possibilities.

____

____

____

____

____

Choose a Solution to Try: After looking at your list of possibilities, which one makes the most sense? What could get in your way when you try out this solution? What are ways you can get over these obstacles?

____

____

____

____

____

How Well Does It Work? Prior to trying out your solution, consider in the end what may make it either successful or unsuccessful. Now try the solution and assess the results. If it didn't work, try one of your other ideas.

____

____

____

____

____

FIGURE 3.2. The ITCH problem-solving sheet for students to complete (based on Muñoz et al., 2000).

support in the problem-solving process. If problematic behaviors, thoughts, or underlying beliefs are playing an active role in the situation, you can then address them with the techniques presented in this and future chapters. The problematic behaviors, thoughts, and/or underlying beliefs can also be established as treatment plan anchors if they are playing an ongoing role in the student's difficulties.

HELPING STUDENTS UNDERSTAND THE COGNITIVE MODEL

Before choosing session anchors—behaviors, thinking patterns, and/or underlying beliefs— you will need to assess the degree to which the student understands the cognitive model. As noted throughout this book, CT is founded on the notion that the way students think about a situation, rather than the situation itself, directly influences the students' emotions. The cognitive model should be described in the first session, using a simple example like the one described in Chapter 1 (the rollercoaster story). That being said, the cognitive model may need to be reviewed throughout counseling, and the narrative that follows demonstrates a way of reviewing the model with students by using a slightly more sophisticated example. The narrative reflects a conversation between a clinician and the student named Michele who was introduced in Chapter 1. Of course, each clinician has a unique personal style, and we encourage you to adapt this cognitive model explanation to the style you already use in counseling. This narrative simply provides an example of one way to present the model. As with the other narratives in this book, this conversation represents a fairly simple conversation, whereas many adolescents may struggle more with the concepts, or be less invested in counseling. The goal of the narrative is to illustrate the overall concept behind presenting the model to a student, rather than including the idiosyncrasies of a real conversation.

> CLINICIAN: Michele, I really appreciate how honest you've been with me about what is happening in your life. I know it can be hard to talk about personal concerns with someone you're just getting to know. I have some ideas about ways that we could really make your life better, but it will take some work on your part to be honest in reflecting on your thoughts, and then practice what we talk about.
>
> MICHELE: OK . . . at this point I'll try anything.
>
> CLINICIAN: Great. Then let's talk some more about the cognitive model. We've already talked a little bit about it as a way of understanding how we all come to think, feel, and act the way we do. We're going to use that model to understand some of the experiences you're going through so we can figure out how to make them be different. Once you are able to use the model, you will be more effective at making yourself feel better. In this model, thoughts (*pointing to head*), not situations themselves, influence the way we feel (*pointing to chest*). For instance, if I woke up this morning and thought, "I'm gonna have a great day today even if it is rainy outside,"

would I feel differently than I would if I thought, "It's rainy again, and it's gonna be another miserable day"?

MICHELE: I guess, but maybe the rain really does just put you in a bad mood or maybe you could have just been in a bad mood.

CLINICIAN: Great point, and we can explore your thoughts more on that. What we've found is that there's actually a thought that comes before the feeling, and the thought is what makes a difference. If we work hard together, I think we can give you some more control over what you think. Do you remember that rollercoaster example we talked about in our first session?

MICHELE: Yeah, and then we did the example of when someone bumps me in the hall, too.

CLINICIAN: Right. Did the idea that it is the thought about the person bumping you, like whether it was an accident or on purpose, and not the bump itself that causes the feeling make sense?

MICHELE: Yeah, but I don't understand how someone can just change a thought. I just think whatever I think!

THOUGHT BUBBLES

Thought bubbles are a great way to make the very abstract idea of "catching thoughts" a little more concrete. Thought bubble activities use cartoon drawings with a "thought bubble" drawn over the head of one or more characters—the way that thoughts are illustrated in a newspaper cartoon. Thought bubbles can be used as one of the many ways to think about thoughts in CT. For example, thought bubbles were used in Chapter 1 to identify the different things Jeremy and Trevor were saying to themselves about the rollercoaster (Figure 1.5). As you can see in Figure 3.3, the thought bubble is fairly straightforward. In this scene, one adolescent is smiling and the other adolescent is frowning. The student is asked to write in the thoughts that each adolescent may be having. Typically, the student will put in a pleasant thought or positive take on the situation in the thought bubble attached to the smiling adolescent and a negative thought or take on the situation in the bubble attached to the frowning adolescent. After the student fills in the thoughts, he or she is then asked to explain why each adolescent, experiencing the same situation, has different feelings. This exercise helps students to think about how the different thoughts, not the situation (which is the same for both cartoon adolescents), are what caused the emotions. Figure 3.3 is an example of a thought bubble activity that may have helped Michele if she had not understood how thinking relates to feelings and situations. Reproducible versions of thought bubble activities are included in Appendices 3.1 and 3.2 at the back of the book for you to copy and use with your students.

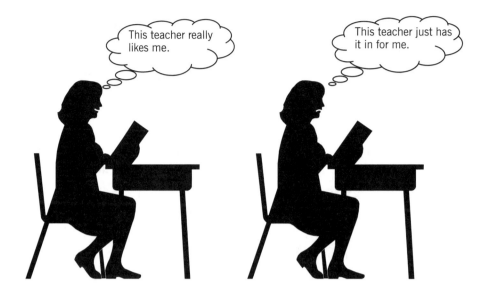

FIGURE 3.3. Thought bubble activity.

Thought bubbles can be used creatively in CT in many different ways, whenever automatic thoughts or images are the topic of conversation. For example, when a student is struggling to identify an automatic thought in a situation, it can be helpful to draw a picture of what was happening in the situation with a thought bubble over the picture of the student and ask the student to fill it in. Another fun exercise is to draw two different cartoons—one with a coping thought in the thought bubble, and another with an unhelpful or inaccurate thought in the thought bubble (see Figure 3.4). These drawings can spur conversation about how the two thoughts would lead to different reactions, helping students understand the power of coping thoughts.

When a student is struggling to identify the automatic thought in a situation, using thought bubble cartoons can also be helpful. Using a three-frame cartoon (Figure 3.5), the situation is drawn in the first frame, the reaction is drawn in the third frame, and then the clinician and student can use the second frame to try out different guesses about what was happening in the middle frame (the automatic thought). Filling in different automatic thoughts can help make sense of the reaction to the situation. You may find many other uses for cartoons and thought bubbles, too, as you work to find a style that fits you and your students. Some clinicians also like to use the idea of thought bubbles with pictures cut from magazines, photos, or other images, asking students to identify what would be in the thought bubble of the person in the picture. Feel free to make your own versions of these activities to meet the needs of your students.

In Figure 3.6, draw a three-frame cartoon based on your strong reaction to a situation you have faced. (These are the situations with the most easily identified automatic thoughts.) In the first frame, draw what was happening in the situation just before your strong reac-

In the first box, draw a situation that includes a character with a thought bubble over his or her head. What is that person saying to him- or herself? Be sure to think about how that thought would lead to that person's feelings or behavior in the situation. In the second box, give that character a different thought in the thought bubble. How did the new thought lead to different feelings or behavior?

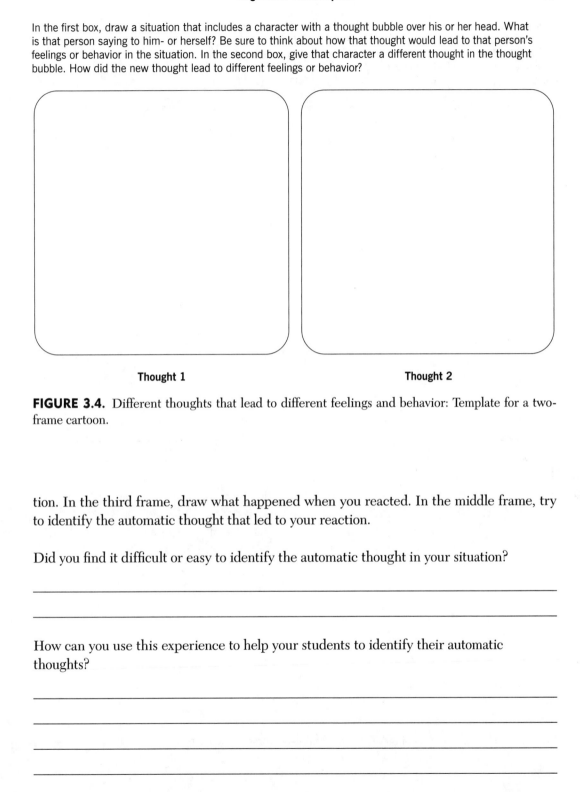

FIGURE 3.4. Different thoughts that lead to different feelings and behavior: Template for a two-frame cartoon.

tion. In the third frame, draw what happened when you reacted. In the middle frame, try to identify the automatic thought that led to your reaction.

Did you find it difficult or easy to identify the automatic thought in your situation?

_____

_____

How can you use this experience to help your students to identify their automatic thoughts?

_____

_____

_____

_____

_____

Below, draw a three-box cartoon that shows how a situation, thought, and reaction are related. In Box 1, draw the situation. What is happening? Who is there? What are they doing? In Box 2, draw a picture that includes a thought bubble. What is the main character's automatic thought in the situation? In Box 3, show the main character's reaction. What is the person feeling? How does the person act?

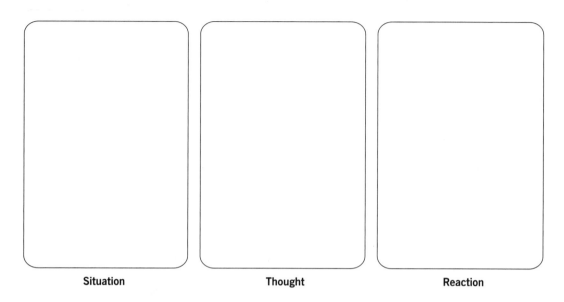

FIGURE 3.5. Template for a three-frame cartoon.

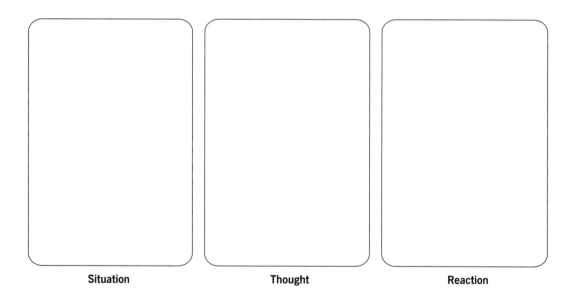

FIGURE 3.6. Three-box practice activity.

THE COGNITIVE TRIANGLE

Another effective way to describe the cognitive model to students is to illustrate the connection between thoughts, behavior, and feelings with the **cognitive triangle** (Clarke, Lewinsohn, & Hops, 1990). The cognitive triangle shows the two-way relationships between thoughts, emotions, and behaviors, and it can be used as a visual aid when you explain the cognitive model to students or refer to it later in counseling. Drawing the cognitive triangle can be particularly helpful with younger adolescents or adolescents with a lower intellectual capacity, because it creates a concrete sense of the connections among thoughts, feelings, and behaviors. Figure 3.7 presents an example of the cognitive triangle that could be used to help Michele understand the connection between her thoughts, feelings, and behavior in specific situations.

In using the cognitive triangle with Michele, we would first show her how thoughts, feelings, and behaviors, which relate to those that she may have, are connected. For example, let's look back at the example from Chapter 1, in which several boys laughed as Michele walked by them in the cafeteria. If we draw the cognitive triangle for Michele, as shown in Figure 3.8, we can show her how the thoughts she had in that situation influenced her feelings and behavior. Next, we would help her develop more helpful or accurate thoughts and explore how those thoughts change her feelings and behavior, as we describe later in this chapter.

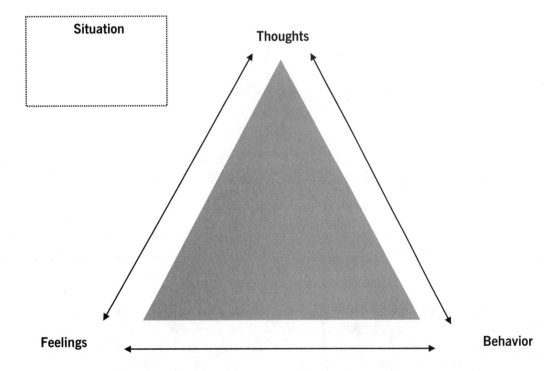

FIGURE 3.7. The cognitive triangle.

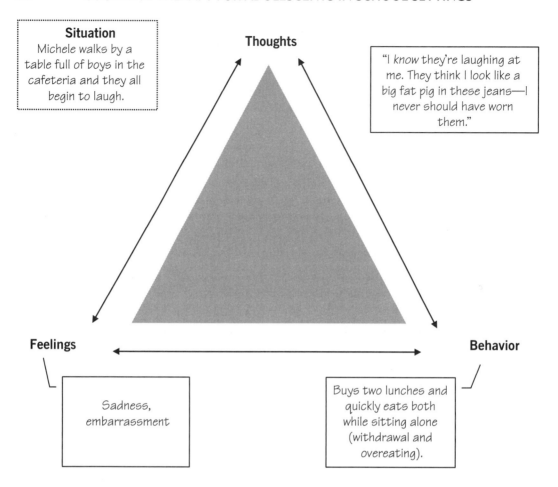

Situation
Michele walks by a table full of boys in the cafeteria and they all begin to laugh.

Thoughts

"I know they're laughing at me. They think I look like a big fat pig in these jeans—I never should have worn them."

Feelings

Sadness, embarrassment

Behavior

Buys two lunches and quickly eats both while sitting alone (withdrawal and overeating).

FIGURE 3.8. Cognitive triangle for Michele.

UNDERSTANDING THE DIFFERENCE BETWEEN THOUGHTS AND EMOTIONS

Many students will initially find it difficult to understand the difference between thoughts and emotions. There are many ways to guide them to an understanding of the difference. A simple starting place is to explain that, "Thoughts are in your head and are usually many words, and emotions are in your body, and they are usually described with one word." Thoughts can also be described as "what you are saying to yourself," while emotions are "what you feel inside." Lower functioning students may need more help understanding this difference, and we suggest keeping an emotion list for reference.

These activities are just a few of the many ways in which you can use your creativity in CT.

Use your creativity to help students recognize their feelings—or to convey any difficult-to-grasp concept in CT! Other activities that we have seen work with students include:

- Flip through magazines together to identify the feelings shown by people in the photos.
- Have the student identify the sensations in his or her body when a strong emotion happens—like butterflies in the stomach and pounding heart for worry, heaviness and slowness for sadness, and so on. Write out a list for reference later.
- Take a walk! Walk with your student through the halls of the school, the cafeteria, or other places full of people. Quietly share with each other the different emotions you see reflected on the faces of others.
- Feelings charades is a fun way to recognize emotions. Brainstorm as many emotions as you can together and write them all on slips of paper. Take turns choosing a slip and act out the emotion until the other person guesses it.
- Have an artistic student draw a picture of himself, illustrating the places in his body where he feels emotions—like sweaty palms, pounding heart, tearful eyes, and so on.
- Anything else that will get the student interested and help her understand and recognize feelings!

Many students will need some combination of the thought bubble activity, cognitive triangle, the emotion list, and other aids to help them understand the cognitive model. As you are teaching them the model, try to be mindful of your use of the word "feeling" to describe "thinking" and vice versa. We have found that many beginning cognitive clinicians use thinking and feeling interchangeably, so be careful to model the correct labeling of feelings and thoughts in session. For example, when a student is beginning CT, he may frequently say things like, "I felt like she was just doing it to be mean." You can then gently restate what he told you with more accurate labels, saying, "So you were thinking (*pointing to your head*) that she was just doing it to be mean. What were you feeling (*pointing to your chest*)?" If the student tells you, "I was feeling like she shouldn't do that!", then review the concepts more explicitly. For example: "Great job of labeling the thought (*pointing to your head*). Remember that feelings usually happen here (*pointing to your chest*) and are usually one word."

It is also important to not force this issue at the expense of the therapeutic relationship when the student is in the middle of sharing an important story. That kind of interruption can feel disrespectful and uncaring to the student. When this occurs, use empathy while the student shares the important part of the story. Then, after you have reflected to the student that you understood him, return to the issue of the difference between thoughts and feelings. Once the student names a feeling, reinforce that skill. For example: "I can see how that thought would hurt. You did a great job of labeling the thought—she was just doing it to be mean, and the feeling—hurt and angry. I would feel hurt, too, if someone were doing something just to be mean to me."

Empathic corrective feedback is a part of the teaching process that helps the student use the cognitive model. We hope that you can see how this kind of feedback can be given warmly and supportively. It is also important to note that the students' feelings are never regarded as wrong or as what needs to be directly changed. Instead, the feeling is always validated, and you will work with students to change the thought so that results their feelings change. Be sure to spend time really listening to students, making sure that you understand what the students are trying to tell you and communicating empathy. After all, it makes sense that students feel bad if they have thinking patterns that lead them to negative feelings—even if the thinking patterns are not based on the evidence. This validation should take place throughout therapy to help strengthen the therapeutic relationship and the resulting traction needed to utilize your cognitive therapy techniques.

THE THOUGHT RECORD

Presenting and explaining the cognitive model can frequently be done in one or two sessions. After the student demonstrates that he or she understand the cognitive model, you can introduce the **thought record** (Beck et al., 1979). The thought record is a great way to demonstrate to students how their situation, thoughts, and feelings relate to one another. The simple version of the thought record guides the student to identify a situation, followed by an automatic thought, which then leads to an emotion. Once the student is comfortable with how to use a thought record and has demonstrated that he or she can do so with little support in session, you can offer encouragement to complete one on another thought for homework. Additional information is gathered for the more complex thought record, adding columns related to challenging automatic thoughts and developing more helpful or accurate thoughts. These more complex thought records are described later in this chapter.

An example of a simple thought record is presented in Figure 3.9, while Figure 3.10 is a partially completed thought record that references what Michele may have written. Reproducible thought records are included in Appendices 3.3 and 3.4 at the end of the

---

SITUATION

What happened around you just before you felt the way you did?

AUTOMATIC THOUGHT(S)

What thought(s) went through your head?

EMOTION(S)

What emotion(s) did you feel—in one word descriptions?

FIGURE 3.9. Simple thought record.

Situation *What happened?*	Thoughts *What thoughts went through my head?*	Feelings *What were my emotions?*	Behaviors *What did I do?*
I walked by a table full of boys in the cafeteria and they all laughed.	I know they're laughing at me. They think I look like a big fat pig in these jeans. I never should have worn them. Besides, I bet Jay told them that we hooked up. I'm sure they think I'm a total slut, too.	Sad, embarrassed	Buy two lunches and ate both as fast as I could while I sat alone.
I sat at an empty table at lunch time to eat.	?	Lonely, sad, hopeless	Withdrew even more and talked to no one for the rest of the day.
I ate too much at dinner, so that my stomach was uncomfortably full.	I have no self-control. I'm going to be fat forever, and no one will ever love me because I'm so fat.	?	Made myself throw up, cried for an hour.
My mother asks me why I don't have a boyfriend right now.	She only wants to know to make sure I won't "steal" her boyfriend again. She doesn't care about me at all—only herself!	Guilty, angry	?

FIGURE 3.10. Fill-in-the-blank thought record example for Michele. Can you take a guess at how Michele might fill in the rest of her thought record?

book. They can be copied for students as they begin to understand the cognitive model and apply it to themselves. As you can see on the thought record form, students can use the questions listed along the left side of the form as a prompt for how to complete the thought record. Listing the situations, thoughts, and emotions in relation to one another reinforces a clear understanding of how thoughts lead to emotions. Using thought records for homework will also help you and the student understand which situations and thoughts are triggering strong emotions outside of counseling sessions. Over time, thought records reveal patterns in your student's thoughts, which inform you about the student's thinking tendencies as well as the situations that trigger thinking patterns.

Look at the thought record in Figure 3.10 and imagine how Michele might complete the sections left "blank." As an example, the record is completed for her thoughts, feelings, and behaviors when she walked into the cafeteria.

GUIDED DISCOVERY

As you may have noticed in the previous role plays and in our descriptions of interventions, the cognitive school clinician rarely, if ever, tells students how they should respond to a situation. In fact, after the first three sessions of cognitive therapy, you will *tell* your students very little about how to make sense of and respond to situations. Instead, you will use what we call **guided discovery** (Burns, 1980). Guided discovery can be very difficult for beginning cognitive clinicians, but it is foundational to effectively using CT techniques.

> **Guided discovery involves asking strategic questions to lead a student to a new perspective.**

Guided discovery is a method of using well-timed and strategic questions to lead students to explore and change inaccurate or unhelpful beliefs, thoughts, and behaviors. For example, guided discovery can be used to look at the evidence that supports or disconfirms the automatic thoughts that students have. This approach is key to checking the thought, which is one of the three steps to changing a thought (presented on p. 71). Our experience with high school students suggests that using the Socratic method or the "Columbo approach" works best when attempting to guide students to a more reasonable or adaptive conclusion. The **Columbo approach** (Selekman, 1993), named after the television show detective who exemplified it, consists of playing a curious, humble, and unassuming questioner so that the student takes the lead in coming to a reasonable conclusion in light of the evidence. As the clinician, you have a clear idea where you are leading the student, but you do so by asking questions that encourage the student to draw her own conclusions, rather than providing the answers yourself. This method encourages students to "own" the answers themselves, rather than seeing them as *your* adult answers. Let's look at the following narrative between Anjanae and her clinician as they use guided discovery.

CLINICIAN: So it sounds like you have been feeling frustrated because you failed your exam.

ANJANAE: Yeah, I can't believe it.

CLINICIAN: I'd really like to hear more about it. I can sure see that you're upset, and I haven't ever heard you mention getting an F before.

ANJANAE: Technically it wasn't an F. But I certainly failed.

CLINICIAN: What was the grade?

ANJANAE: I got a B, and that is failing to me.

CLINICIAN: OK, I see. I can understand that failing would be really hard for you, and I can also see where high standards like that could make a lot of people feel frustrated.

ANJANAE: Yes, this happens all the time.

CLINICIAN: All the time?

ANJANAE: Well, not all the time. I guess this is actually the first time this semester.

CLINICIAN: So . . . it sounds like this is the first time you have not received an A this semester, and that feels really bad.

ANJANAE: Yeah, and I guess, when you say it that way, it doesn't seem so bad.

CLINICIAN: You said, "It doesn't seem so bad."

ANJANAE: Well, yeah, I actually kind of feel stupid for reacting this way . . . but I can't help it. I kind of think I'm overreacting when I think about it, but I still feel really upset.

CLINICIAN: I think that it makes sense that you feel bad, but is this about you being stupid or failing, or more about your high standards?

ANJANAE: What do you mean?

CLINICIAN: Well, is someone who receives all A's with one exception "stupid"?

ANJANAE: No, I guess I just really have high standards.

CLINICIAN: So you have high standards, and what are these doing for you?

ANJANAE: Helping me achieve, but when I don't, I feel horrible.

CLINICIAN: So I wonder what might make more sense for you?

ANJANAE: Keeping my high standards, but maybe easing up on myself when I inevitably don't meet them every once and a while.

CLINICIAN: That seems like it could help.

The clinician would then praise Anjanae for being so open to examining her thinking and encourage her to apply one of the techniques listed in this chapter or Chapter 4 to change her thinking. The clinician would also make a note of the thinking traps that Anjanae tends to use (like Shoulds or A Perfect Disaster from Chapter 1), which could be addressed in future sessions as they continue to pop up. The clinician would also keep track of Anjanae's intermediate belief that she has to be perfect and high achieving to be capable and incorporate it into her cognitive conceptualization of Anjanae.

THE THREE C'S

Using guided discovery with students in early sessions frequently sets the stage for helping students identify and evaluate thoughts. In doing so, students learn to see you as someone who will not to lecture them, and they see your office as a place where

> The Three C's—catch, check, change—are key techniques for students to master.

they will not be told what to do or that what they are doing is wrong. Guiding the student to an understanding of his or her unhelpful or inaccurate thoughts and healthy replacement thoughts frequently flows through a process that can be described in three steps—the **Three C's** (Granholm, McQuaid, Auslander, & McClure, 2004; Granholm, et al., 2005). The Three C's are a logical outgrowth of the cognitive model and the simple thought record. In many cases, you will be able to use the Three C's to help students work through their problematic thinking patterns. In fact, the Three C's will frequently be the therapeutic framework for the majority of cognitive techniques you will use while doing cognitive counseling. While guiding the student through the Three C's, you will be asking her to identify the thought that came before her emotion (catching), reflect on how accurate and useful the thought is (checking), and then change the thought to a more helpful or accurate one as needed (changing).

One way to help students understand this process, particularly when working with students who think more concretely, is to compare it to being a detective. Together, you will track down the evidence for or against different thoughts so that the student can make decisions about which thoughts are the most accurate and helpful for them. We used detective language in many of the examples that follow, to demonstrate how the techniques can be described. However, as with other techniques in CT, you should trust your clinical judgment and feedback from students to decide which students will respond well to a detective analogy and which students will prefer a different kind of description. The following pages detail the steps of the Three C's and suggest ways to effectively apply them in schools.

Catching

The first step in helping a student modify thinking patterns is **catching** (Granholm, 2004; 2005), or identifying the thought that occurred just before the student experienced a negative emotion. This skill was already introduced when the student completed a thought record and identified the thought that followed the triggering situation and preceded the emotion. While learning this skill, the thought is often not caught until after the situation, when the student and clinician work back through what happened when the student felt bad and identified the thought that came before the emotion. You can do this by asking something like, "Just before you felt angry, what words or pictures went through your head? What did you say to yourself?" When the thought is identified, the student will also rate how strongly he believes the thought (often rated as believing it from 0 to 100%). This rating serves two purposes: it guides the student to think about the shades of gray between believing and not believing a thought, and it gives a basis against which to measure any changes in the strength of his belief in the thought as a result of the Three C's. Once the student is skilled at catching thoughts, he will become able to recognize the thought as it occurs and understand that this thought is what led to the emotion. The following example illustrates one way this intervention may play out in session.

CLINICIAN: Remember the other day when I described the cognitive model?

DAVID: Yeah, it says that it is not the situation that causes my feelings . . . it is my thoughts about the situation.

CLINICIAN: Exactly. Good memory, David. Along with this, I mentioned that we will work together to change some of the thinking that leads you to feel so bad, using a technique called the Three C's. The Three C's have three steps called catching, checking, and changing.

DAVID: OK . . .

CLINICIAN: The first step, catching, is what you already are doing when you identify, or catch, the thought that comes before an emotion. The second step is called checking, and when you do this you are checking the thought for two things—whether the thought is *accurate* and *useful*.

DAVID: So I'm trying to see if the thought is true and if it is helpful? What if it's not that helpful or true?

CLINICIAN: Good question. . . . That is when you'll change the thought. We can go over ways to do that after we practice the first two steps—catching and checking.

DAVID: Uh huh. And what if the thought really is true? Not all of my thoughts can be wrong, can they?

CLINICIAN: I'm really glad you asked that. Cognitive therapy really isn't about just glossing over things or just thinking a happy thought—it is about being more accurate at seeing what is what. We'll be a lot like detectives, gathering evidence for and against some thoughts. Sometimes the evidence will show that the thought is probably true, and sometimes it will show the thought is probably not true. If the thought might be true but isn't that helpful to you, or it just isn't true, we'll look at ways to think differently about things. Are you willing to give this a try and see what you think?

DAVID: Sure, I guess so.

The clinician would invite David to apply "catching" to a situation that he commonly encounters or has recently experienced until he demonstrates a good grasp of the skill. Catching would then be followed by checking and changing, as we present in the following pages. For this and all CT skills, we suggest first demonstrating the skills for students, then practicing them together with students, and then having students practice the skills themselves. These steps are outlined below (Moats & Hall, 1999):

1. I (the clinician) do.
2. We (the clinician and student together) do.
3. You (the student tries it himself in session) do.

In teaching these steps, do not move on to the next step until the student has mastered the previous step. It is very important that the student experiences a sense of mastery of each technique in session, because without this feeling, she may leave the session more stressed and unlikely to practice techniques in between sessions.

Checking

The second C, **checking** the thought, involves determining whether the thought is accurate and helpful for the student, and this can only be done after the thought is caught (Granholm et al., 2004; 2005). While in session, you can also use the catching and checking techniques when you or the student notice that she experiences a strong negative feeling. This is called catching and checking a **hot thought** (Beck, 1995), because it is done when the thought is hot, or in the front of the student's mind. Catching a hot thought in session overlaps in some ways with what is conceptualized in other therapies as focusing on the therapeutic process. Doing so can strengthen the therapeutic alliance, as well as address problematic thinking patterns that play out in session. For instance, upon seeing a student frown, you may say something like, "David, I noticed your frown when we talked about cutting our meetings from two times a week to once a week." Following this, the clinician should then encourage the student to go through the first two C's in session. First, the student would identify the thought that came before the feeling (catching). Then, the student would check to see how thoughtful and accurate the thought was. There are a number of techniques for checking the thought, which we will introduce below.

Questions to Ask When Checking a Thought

The questions the student will use when checking a thought are listed on the Three C's thought record (Granholm et al., 2004, 2005). The Three C's thought record builds on what the student learned with the simple thought record: how to identify a thought in relation to both a situation and an emotion. The the Three C's thought record adds checking and changing the thought, after it is caught. After students have mastered these skills and can complete the Three C's thought record in session, it can be assigned as homework. (A reproducible version can be found in Appendix 3.5 at the back of the book.) This sheet will become a mainstay in students' toolboxes of techniques that will help them identify their thinking traps and more helpful/accurate thoughts or responses.

The Three C's thought record has some questions listed on it to help the student work through the process. Other helpful questions (Beck, 1995) are listed below. A reproducible version of these questions is included in Appendix 3.6. We recommend that you use questions like these in sessions to help students understand how to check their thoughts.

- "What tells you that this thought is true? What tells you that it might not be true?" (For students using the detective analogy, these questions may be: "What is the evidence that this thought is true? Not true?")
- "Is there another explanation for what happened?"
- "What is the impact of your believing this thought?" (pros/cons)
- "What should you do about it?"
- "If this happened to a friend, what would you tell him or her?"
- "What would your friends say about your thoughts?"
- "Is this thought helpful?"

When the thought that is being evaluated is related to anxiety, students typically fear that something bad is going to happen. To evaluate an anxiety thought, the following questions may also be helpful (Beck, 1995):

- "What is the worst thing that could happen?" (This is typically the main question that students dwell on when they worry.)
- "What is the best thing that could happen?"
- "What is the most likely thing to happen?"
- "If the worst thing happened, could you deal with it?"

In the following narrative, David and his clinician use some of the techniques just described to catch, check, and change a thought (Granholm et al., 2004, 2005).

CLINICIAN: David, I noticed a frown when we talked about cutting our meetings from two times a week to once a week.

DAVID: Yeah, that sucks. I don't feel that great about it.

CLINICIAN: Thanks for telling me, David. Your honesty is always really helpful. Let's apply the Three C's to this and see if we can't get a better grasp on what's going on. What thought went through your head right after I said we should cut back to one session a week?

DAVID: I was mad.

CLINICIAN: Good identification of a feeling—mad. What thoughts went through your head?

DAVID: You don't want to see me as much as you have been because you don't like me.

CLINICIAN: Great work, David. You just caught the thought. How much do you believe that thought?

DAVID: 90%.

CLINICIAN: OK. Let's check it. Is it accurate? And is it useful?

DAVID: Well I'm not sure . . . I remember you said that I need to check the evidence to see if a thought is accurate.

CLINICIAN: Exactly. So what in the situation suggested that I don't like you and what suggests that I do like you? [If the student is unable to think of reasons on either side of the "argument," having the student brainstorm all the possibilities, write them down, and then choose the most likely from the list can be helpful.]

DAVID: Well, you smile when you see me, you make time in your day to see me, and you have said on lots of occasions that I am doing good work here. But . . . you are cutting back your time for me.

CLINICIAN: OK, good. What is the most reasonable explanation for my suggesting that we cut back time together? [Again, encourage brainstorming if necessary.]

DAVID: That I'm making progress. . . . Hmm, I guess when I look at it like that, it seems more reasonable that you cut back because I am doing better.

CLINICIAN: You just completed the steps to changing that thought! Good work, David. Now how strongly do you believe your first thought that I don't like you?

DAVID: 40%.

CLINICIAN: That's a big change! Well, I think there is a lot of evidence saying that I do like you. And I know that you said that your first thought made you feel mad. How do you feel now?

DAVID: Not as mad. I guess I mostly feel proud because you and I both think I'm making progress. I feel a little nervous, too, because I'm not sure once a week is enough.

CLINICIAN: I think that this was a good example of how changing your thought can change your emotion. Nice work! I wonder if we could do the same thing and check out the evidence for your thought about once a week not being enough, since it's leaving you feeling nervous. Want to try it and see what happens?

In this example, the clinician asked the student to rate the strength of the belief they were checking before and after he changed it. This example can also be applied to emotions by asking the student to rate the intensity of the emotion before and after he or she changes the related thought. These ratings help the student recognize how the Three C's affect thinking and feeling so that the student is more likely to use this strategy out of session.

The previous narrative between David and his clinician was an example of the Three C's catching, checking, and changing taking place, one after the other. While this can and will occur, the processes of checking and changing may need to be explicitly taught before the student can apply it the way David did. The process of **changing** thoughts, the third step, will be explicitly described later in the chapter but when the student does it naturally, as in the dialogue above, she or he should be applauded for doing so. Also, when the student does this in session, it will frequently increase his or her motivation and investment in therapy. The following dialogue represents a conversation between Michele and her clinician that could take place after the Three C's were reviewed.

> CLINICIAN: Michele, let's look at the thought that you just caught, "He is disgusted by me," because I think you will notice some important things. Let's try checking that thought. As we talked about last session, when checking your thought you need to ask yourself two questions: Is the thought accurate? And is the thought working for me?
>
> MICHELE: OK. But I really do think he was disgusted by me.
>
> CLINICIAN: How much do you believe that?
>
> MICHELE: 100%.
>
> CLINICIAN: All right, well, you will always start with looking at whether the thought is accurate. What evidence suggested that your thought was true?
>
> MICHELE: Well he just glanced at me and then looked away.

The clinician in this situation could then help Michele check the thought with a number of different techniques. For example, Michele could (1) check the evidence for and against her thought; (2) consider other explanations for the person glancing at her and then looking away; or (3) consider what a friend would say to her about what happened or what she would say to a friend in the same situation. Let's look at each of these options in more detail.

1. **Checking the evidence** involves just what it sounds like—checking whether the student's thought is supported by the evidence that was in the situation. One way to introduce this to a student is by asking what there is about the situation that supports the thought and what there is about it that does not. The student should then list all of the evidence for and against her thought. It is important that the student list *all* of the evidence she has for and

against her thought. Otherwise, challenging her thought will not be as effective, because the student may be holding some "yes, but" kinds of thoughts in her mind that could undermine the Three C process. After examining the evidence, she is then asked to indicate how strongly she still believes her original thought. If the original thought no longer seems entirely accurate, the student is encouraged to find a more reasonable alternative thought, which is a thought that reflects the evidence, or an **adaptive response** thought, which is a thought that follows her negative automatic thought. The adaptive response thought is something she can tack on to her negative automatic thought to make it more reasonable.

For lower functioning students or more concrete thinkers, we have used a dialogue similar to the following. "If I told you I had 10 desks in my office, would you believe me?" After the student says no, you ask her how she knew that the statement was not true. Have the student describe the process she engaged in when checking the evidence, which involved looking around the office and seeing only one desk. The student is praised for "checking" the evidence and then encouraged to apply this process to her automatic thoughts and beliefs.

2. **Considering alternative explanations** involves looking at other ways to explain situations and the behaviors of others. Often, students will have an automatic thought involving a thinking trap without considering more realistic explanations. We encourage students to write out their initial explanation for an event, and then list all other possible explanations. Each explanation is rated based on how likely it is to be true, or the likelihood is mapped out in a pie chart like the one in Figure 3.11. In our experience, when students see all of the alternative explanations written out on a pie chart, they are often able to quickly see that their initial thought may not be as believable as they first thought.

3. **Considering "What would your friend say?"** requires students to question the accuracy of their thought by taking the perspective of a respected peer and applying the peer's response to their situation. You might ask, "What would Cathy (a peer respected by the student) say about this situation?" or "What would you say to Cathy if she were in your situation?" The clinician would use guided discovery to help the student develop a replacement thought or an adaptive response. Students often find it easier to develop a replacement thought in this less personal way, for a friend, than for themselves.

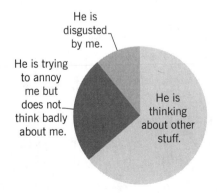

FIGURE 3.11. How likely is each explanation?

The following is a continuation of Michele's conversation with her clinician, showing how guided discovery and considering alternative explanations can be used in the checking step of the Three C's (Granholm et al., 2004, 2005). This conversation also shows how the first two C's lead into changing the thought described on page 76.

MICHELE: Well, he just glanced at me and then looked away.

CLINICIAN: And how did you feel when that happened?

MICHELE: Like a loser.

CLINICIAN: It sounds like that was a really hard thing to have happen. I wonder if he has ever glanced at other people and looked away thinking other things than being disgusted by them? Or maybe not even thought about the person he glanced at?

MICHELE: I don't know what he's thinking about them, but I know what he was thinking when he glanced at me.

CLINICIAN: OK, so if you don't know what he is thinking when he is looking at other people, how do you know what he is thinking when he is looking at you?

MICHELE: I guess I'm not technically really, *really* sure in either case.

CLINICIAN: If you're not sure, is it possible that you may be assuming the worst or incorrectly mind reading?

MICHELE: Maybe.

CLINICIAN: How likely do you think that is? I'm remembering some of the other times where we figured out that you have a tendency to end up in thinking traps like reading minds and jumping to conclusions.

MICHELE: Well, when you say it that way, maybe I was assuming the worst.

CLINICIAN: If you're going to give "assuming the worst" some time in your head, maybe we should also give "assuming what is likely" some time?

MICHELE: Makes sense.

CLINICIAN: OK, so what is likely?

MICHELE: That he did not really even think about me in that moment. That he probably was thinking about other stuff.

Did you notice how the clinician used guided discovery in the above? At this point the clinician would encourage Michele to write down her alternative/more likely explanations and then chart them in a pie diagram.

CLINICIAN: Now that you have all of these explanations charted out, I see that your first explanation only takes a fifth of the chart. Right now, how much do you believe the thought "He was disgusted by me"?

MICHELE: Maybe 20%.

CLINICIAN: Wow, that's an 80% decrease in how much you believed that! And you said you felt pretty bad when that happened with him. Thinking about it now, how do you feel?

MICHELE: Not that bad at all. I mean, if he was thinking about something else, why would that bother me? I feel OK about it now.

CLINICIAN: So what do you think it would do to your negative feelings if you were to think through this kind of process in the future?

MICHELE: If my negative thought seemed less strong, I probably wouldn't feel as bad, either.

CLINICIAN: Great work, Michele.

Considering Whether a Thought Is Helpful

Although we've spent a lot of time working on how to handle thoughts that are not completely accurate, sometimes students have thoughts that are accurate *and* distressing. When this happens, the next step is to check whether the thought is helping the student. In doing so, you will want to encourage a student to consider how helpful it is to continue allowing the thought to be active in the front of his or her mind. The following is an example of a conversation between a clinician and David, where David's automatic thought is accurate, distressing, and as a result, not helpful for him.

CLINICIAN: So, it sounds like one of the things that contributes to your stress is that you're finding yourself in class thinking, "I will *never* be able to read as fast as the rest of the people in this class."

DAVID: Yeah, and I won't ever read as fast. I'm a really slow reader because of my learning disorder.

CLINICIAN: Well for starters, you did a good job of catching the thought, "I will never be able to read as fast as the rest of the people in this class." Let's move to checking it . . . and remember that checking consists of two steps which include . . .

DAVID: Is the thought accurate and is the thought working for me. The thought is accurate . . .

CLINICIAN: So, is it helpful for you to think, "I will never be able to read as fast as the rest of the people in this class," and to think about that all during class?

DAVID: No, I guess not. I just end up feeling worse and worse the longer I think about it, and I just want to give up and go hang out in the cafeteria. It sucks.

CLINICIAN: I can see where that would suck. Good work though . . . you just checked it, and now let's work on changing it—because it is not working for you.

DAVID: OK.

The clinician and student would then move to the next step in the Three C's: changing. After the student has a good grasp of the first two steps, you can assign homework to practice the technique out of session.

Changing

Changing thoughts (Granholm et al., 2004, 2005), the third step, often flows naturally out of the checking step, as it did in the previous narratives with David and Michele. There are many strategies for changing thoughts, but the strategies that are most commonly used in schools are the behavioral strategies (presented in Chapter 4) and cognitive strategies that lead to replacement thoughts and adaptive responses.

A replacement thought replaces a student's inaccurate or unhelpful thought with a thought that is either more accurate than his previous thought, directly challenging of it, or a soothing take on the thought. Most often, these thoughts are developed during guided discovery, after the student recognizes automatic thoughts that are unhelpful or inaccurate. Through continued guided discovery, you will be able to help the student explore thoughts that are more accurate

> **Replacement thoughts are *not* just thinking a happy thought! Help students develop thoughts that are believable and in their own words.**

and helpful. The most important feature of a good replacement thought is that it be one that feels believable to the student—not just a "happy thought." The replacement thought should also be in the student's own words and should be short enough to be quickly said. After developing a replacement thought, you will want to encourage your students to practice using it out of sessions. Let him know that using the replacement thought may be difficult at first, but that the more he practices using the new thought, the better he will become at replacing his negative thoughts. You can use the analogy of riding a bike: "When you first learned to ride a bike, the more you did it, the easier it became. Replacement thoughts work the same way. The more you use your replacement thought, the better you will become at using it. After using the replacement thought for a while, it will become automatic, and you won't have to think about it, just as riding a bike gets to be automatic after a while." With enough practice, the replacement thought will become an automatic thought.

COPING CARDS

We recommend that you write down techniques used in session with the student so that she can review them when out of session. One way to do this involves **coping cards** (Beck, 1995), which can be used to help students evaluate their automatic thoughts and activate or motivate themselves to work towards short- and long-term goals. Let's look first at coping cards that can be used to evaluate automatic thoughts.

A student may need to use an adaptive response thought that tacks on to an automatic unhelpful or inaccurate thought. For instance, a student who is accidentally bumped by another student in the hall may automatically think, "He is trying to mess with me!", even after having done guided discovery work about whether these kinds of automatic thoughts are always accurate (or helpful). Instead of expecting the student to have the immediate automatic thought of, "The hallway is crowded, so that was probably an accident," he should be initially encouraged to work on an adaptive response to follow the automatic thought like, "He is trying to mess with me! . . . I'm assuming the worst and he is probably just trying to get to where he needs to go and accidentally bumped into me."

Coping cards are collaboratively created by the student and clinician to offer helpful responses to situations and thoughts. For example, when David first came to your office, one of the first things he said was that he was "never good enough and never fit in." After 2 months of working with David, you and he notice that these thoughts often pop into his head when he goes to his "default setting" of thinking of himself as a failure and an oddball, of feeling sad, and of withdrawing from situations. In one session, you and he develop an adaptive response thought to cope with his automatic thought: "I don't always fit in, but neither did many of the great actors when they were in high school, and what makes me different also makes me unique in a good way." David writes out the automatic thought and his adaptive response on a piece of paper and tucks this adaptive response coping card into his wallet. He also saves a note for himself on his cell phone with the helpful thought. In fact, David could store copies of his adaptive response card anywhere it would be easy for him to remember and access them: his dresser drawer, his e-mail, or his backpack, for example. In the beginning stage of challenging thoughts outside of sessions, each time he catches himself thinking, "I am never good enough. I never fit in," he will pull out and read his helpful thought. Remember that this is more than just "thinking happy thoughts" or a generic affirmation.

Coping cards can also be designed to help students cope with specific problems. Alfred and his clinician found that he frequently has automatic thoughts like, "I'm gonna take that guy down before he can mess with me," when he is bumped in the hall. After he and the clinician identified this thought, the clinician could help Alfred to change the thought and his reaction by creating coping cards. For example, the coping cards in Figures 3.12 and 3.13 are intended to provide Alfred with an adaptive response for his automatic thought (Figure 3.12) and a reminder of his reasons to use his adaptive response (Figure 3.13).

As the clinician and Alfred continue working together, Alfred mentions that he would like to return to the wrestling team, but he believes that "the coach will never let me back onto the team; I've been gone from practices too long." Although this thought may be true,

---

My Automatic Thought: "I 'm gonna take that guy down before he can mess with me."

Adaptive Response: "I need to slow down and think, because when I am in school, it is different from when I am on the streets. There are different rules here, and I want to show my brother how to be a successful man in both places. Just walk away!"

FIGURE 3.12. Adaptive response card.

Why Stop and Think Before I Throw a Punch?

- I can teach my little brother a better way of dealing with life.
- I can get back on the wrestling team and hopefully get a scholarship out of here.
- Reacting gets me in trouble, and these guys aren't worth that.
- There are different rules in school and in the streets, and if I want to get out of here I need to play the game in both of them.
- I need to show my brother how to be successful in school and in life.
- Remember to ask myself—is this problem worth losing my ticket out of here?

FIGURE 3.13. Coping card: Reasons to stop and think.

Alfred is *assuming* that it is true without testing it out, and is therefore not planning to even try to return to the team. Recognizing this, the clinician and Alfred make a plan for a way in which Alfred can check his negative assumption about the coach. This type of **activation/motivation card** can be particularly helpful when a student has a goal that feels too large, complicated, or intimidating to take on.

To develop an activation/motivation card, you will work with the student to clearly define the goal. Next, help the student to think through each of the steps that would lead to reaching that goal. The steps should be concrete, observable, and manageable. Keeping each of the steps manageable so that they can be achieved and crossed off the list helps students feel like their goals are reachable, rather than overwhelming. Any potential barriers should be identified, and coping strategies or problem solving should be planned for managing the barriers. Alfred created an activation/motivation card that looked like Figure 3.14.

With continued practice, Alfred will internalize the replacement thoughts and may even subsequently begin to chip away at underlying beliefs. As he continues to use these cards (or the note on his cell phone, etc.) to remember his more helpful ways of thinking, the replacement thoughts will become more natural to him and ultimately the cards may no longer be necessary. Further, as Alfred's underlying belief about the world changes to one that allows him to trust some people and feel safe in nondangerous situations, and as he demonstrates a less aggressive behavior pattern, the clinician will transition into the last stage of counseling which is described in Chapter 5. The last stage of counseling focuses on strengthening coping skills and relapse prevention.

Plan for Getting Back onto the Wrestling Team

- Remind myself that I'm being a strong man by going back to the team instead of walking away.
- Role-play what I want to say to the coach with my clinician.
- Schedule a private meeting with the coach.
- Tell the coach how I will handle problems with teammates better in the future.
- Practice better anger management skills with my clinician.
- Check in with coach on what I can do better every week and then follow through with it.

FIGURE 3.14. Coping card: Instructions to activate/motivate.

Steps for Finishing Ninth Grade

- Figure out my due date so that I can find out when it falls in the school year.
- Let my teachers know that I will be out of school for health reasons around that time.
- Ask my teachers if there is work I can do before the baby comes so I can stay ahead.
- Make a schedule to plan the schoolwork I need to complete before the baby comes and include a plan for how long I will be out for the baby.
- Find out if there is any help I can get from tutors or if I can get some of my work waived.
- Check my progress on the schedule at the end of each week.
- After I have the baby, check with my teachers every 2 weeks to see what I need to do to stay on track to pass ninth grade and add those things to the schedule.
- Remind myself that I can do this for me and for my baby!!!

FIGURE 3.15. Coping card: Steps for reaching a goal.

Coping cards designed to activate or motivate a student will look very different depending on the needs of the student. Anjanae, for example, might make good use of a coping strategy card. One of her goals is to graduate from high school and college, while also raising her baby. This goal is quite ambitious, so breaking it down into more manageable steps would make planning more feasible. Anjanae decided that her immediate goal is to finish the school year while delivering and keeping the baby, so her clinician suggests that they plan ways to help her to finish ninth grade. Finishing the rest of high school, and then college, are goals that they can also plan together, but creating one detailed plan for all of those long-term goals would probably be overwhelming. These cards can be supplemented by behavioral strategies that will be described in Chapter 4. Anjanae and her clinician might map out a coping strategy card that would look like Figure 3.15.

This coping card includes more than enough steps for now—trying to plan her way through high school and college, all on one card, would be really unmanageable, and would most likely leave Anjanae feeling more overwhelmed than when she started the counseling session. However, planning reasonable steps like the ones above can help students to feel that even large problems can be broken down and tackled step by step. Another card with long-term goals can also help Anjanae feel that she is keeping her long-term focus along with these more immediate goals. Students like Anjanae will also develop a sense of mastery as they are able to check off the steps that they complete and can reinforce themselves for doing so.

ROAD MAP TO SUCCESS

We have referenced some fairly high functioning students in this book, but students can show a really wide range of functioning levels and abilities. Students may struggle with certain CT concepts, be reluctant to write, be particularly drawn to creative outlets, or have other reasons that may require you to modify your techniques. With lower functioning students or students who have a more creative flair, you can modify many techniques by incorporating drawing activities. We have found a drawing exercise called **road map to success** to be very effective in helping students identify the steps to meeting their goals, as Anjanae did when she wrote her goals out on a coping card (Figure 3.16). Rather than writing out a list of goals, the student maps out goals on a colorful map that can be started in session and completed outside of the session for homework. When creating a road map to success, instruct the student to first list with you her short-term (1 week, 2 week, 1 month) goals as well as her long-term (6-month, 1-year, end-of-high-school, etc.) goals. After she has identi-fied her short- and long-term goals, you can work with her to identify obstacles or detours that reflect her treatment anchors such as assuming the worst (thinking pattern anchor) or drinking alcohol (behavior pattern anchor). Finally, check in about how the student will deal with the obstacles by asking about and listing coping strategies—using the Three C's, cop-ing cards, or any behavioral strategies.

The goals can then be depicted on the map by students, with pictures of themselves as they accomplish each goal, along with pictures of themselves running into detours where they may go off the road to success. Students may draw these pictures, illustrate them with clippings from magazines, take photos of themselves acting out the different situations, or use any other method that engages the student in the process. Coping strategies can be listed in a box on the side of the map, as a reference to all of the skills they have to deal with life's challenges. We included an example of what Anjanae may have created with her clinician.

There are countless ways that the road map can look, and even more ways that this idea can be modified. The road map is just one of the many ways that the principles in this book can be modified to engage your students. Enjoy the creativity in these exercises, and both you and your students will be able to have fun in these sessions. A blank road map form is included in Appendix 3.7 at the end of the book, and you can use it as a jumping-off point for your own work.

WHAT TO DO WHEN THE STUDENT CAN'T CHECK OR CHANGE A THOUGHT

We suggest that when a student is struggling to make progress in CT . . . you just give up and schedule a new student to give it a try. Wait—what? Of course, we would never really sug-gest that you give up. Instead, using humor, as we are attempting to do here, is encouraged with students who seem stuck, and it is something we use when training school clinicians, who may need a brief break from the difficult task of learning CT or helping their students. Of course, the effective use of humor is part of each clinician's own therapeutic style, and clinicians will vary in how often or well they use humor. Be aware of your own style and strengths, and remember to relax enough to use humor as appropriate. At the same time, be aware of the student's interpersonal style and your conceptualization, being sure to use humor only to the degree that it is helpful for the student.

When students really do seem stuck, an important question is *why* they are stuck. Some possibilities include:

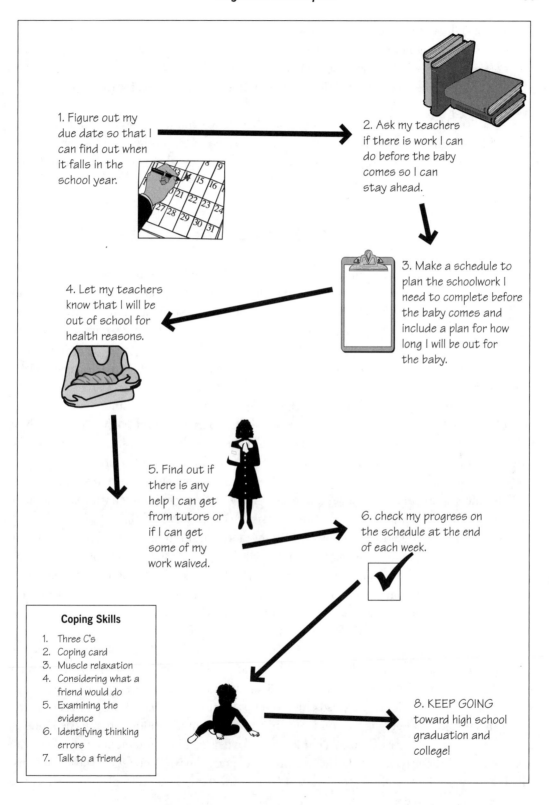

1. Figure out my due date so that I can find out when it falls in the school year.

2. Ask my teachers if there is work I can do before the baby comes so I can stay ahead.

3. Make a schedule to plan the schoolwork I need to complete before the baby comes and include a plan for how long I will be out for the baby.

4. Let my teachers know that I will be out of school for health reasons.

5. Find out if there is any help I can get from tutors or if I can get some of my work waived.

6. check my progress on the schedule at the end of each week.

8. KEEP GOING toward high school graduation and college!

Coping Skills

1. Three C's
2. Coping card
3. Muscle relaxation
4. Considering what a friend would do
5. Examining the evidence
6. Identifying thinking errors
7. Talk to a friend

FIGURE 3.16. Anjanae's road map to success.

- Is a skill or ability deficit is getting in the way?
- Is the student not invested in therapy?
- Has the student developed some resistance?
- Are the concepts being explained in a way that is too complex for the student?

This list represents the main reasons that may leave you and a student feeling stuck. Each of the reasons would lead to a very different way of intervening. The following pages depict ways in which cognitive clinicians can conceptualize what is causing you and your students to get stuck and how to intervene.

REVERSE ROLE PLAY

Some students may be reluctant to work with a school clinician because they assume (have an automatic thought) that the clinician will be like other staff members or authority figures who may not have helped them in the past. In other cases, students may be struggling to understand CT concepts because of emotional or intellectual challenges or because concepts were introduced in a way that was too complicated for them to grasp. To gain a better understanding of what is getting in the way of therapeutic progress, try using a **reverse role play** (Beck et al., 1993).

In a reverse role play, you will invite the student to be the clinician and you will assume the role of the student. Encourage the student to sit in your chair, and ask him to do his best job of being you—a clinician. You can then begin the role play as the student, reciting the thinking patterns that he could not previously identify or alter or whichever other issues had the student stuck. The student's responses, role-playing as you, can be very revealing. If the student states appropriate responses and can identify and alter thinking patterns, it is likely that a skill deficit is not getting in the way—resistance may be the culprit.

Resistance can be addressed by identifying and questioning the student's automatic thoughts and subsequently altering your approach. If the student role-plays an exaggerated version of your style (or an accurate, if uncomfortable version!), be open to this feedback and use it to modify your approach. Skill deficits can be approached by using alternative approaches for presenting the information. This is another opportunity to use your creativity to engage your students in different ways.

While working with adolescents in juvenile correctional facilities, we have found the reverse role play to be especially useful with students who have an oppositional behavior pattern and frequently come to counseling with automatic thoughts like, "I'm not gonna play your game." These students may also enjoy the power shift that occurs when they become the clinician and you become the student. This process can be fun for you and the student, as they adopt a caricature of you as a clinician, and we often hear statements like "Well, you need to change the way you think before you can change the way you feel!" These students, just like yours, will appreciate the praise that follows the reverse role play, as well as the changes you make in counseling to address what you learn from the role play.

RESISTANCE IN COGNITIVE THERAPY

Resistance is understood by CT clinicians to be directly related to the thoughts the students have about the clinician, the therapeutic process, and/or themselves. To address this, you can ask a student in session, "What is going through your mind?" when you sense resistance. If you have a hunch that the resistance may be related to her thoughts about the therapeutic process, you can ask, "What could I do differently to make this more helpful for you?" or "What thoughts do you have about coming here or about what we are doing?" If you think the resistance may relate to worry about disclosing information to you, you could say something like, "What could I as a clinician do with you to help in understanding that anything you say is OK and that I can actually help?" If you suspect that the student's automatic thoughts about herself are getting in the way, you could say something like, "What kinds of things could be hard for a student to talk about in here?" Any of these statements could be prefaced with a statement like, "I really appreciate your coming here today, and I was hoping you could help me understand something about what it's like for students who come to this office. I'd like to ask you some questions, and I really want you to know that whatever you say is OK."

IDENTIFYING AND CHANGING UNDERLYING BELIEFS

The techniques presented in this chapter directly target the thinking patterns that interfere with students reaching their goals. Although these techniques are very effective at changing thinking patterns, they may also be indirectly chipping away at the negative underlying beliefs that feed these thoughts. As students change their behaviors and thoughts and as more positive experiences follow, they will develop a greater sense of self-efficacy and a more realistic and positive view of themselves. We have described this process to students and school clinicians using the air, land, water analogy.

The **air, land, water analogy** describes changes in underlying beliefs as a process that relates to changes in thinking patterns and behaviors (Cory Newman, PhD, personal communication, May 3, 2010). Just as air on a hot summer day changes more quickly than the ground underneath it, so do behavior patterns change more quickly than thinking patterns. The continual changes in behavior patterns then can result in changes in thinking patterns. And, just as it takes a summer of hot days to warm the lake or ocean, so does it take months of changing thinking and behavior patterns for underlying beliefs to change. (See Figure 3.17.) We may explain this to Anjanae in the following way.

CLINICIAN: Anjanae, what changes first on a hot summer day: the air or the ground under your feet?

ANJANAE: Well, it gets hot around noon, so the air's hot, but it takes a while for the ground to catch up. The ground does not warm up until it has been warm for most of the day.

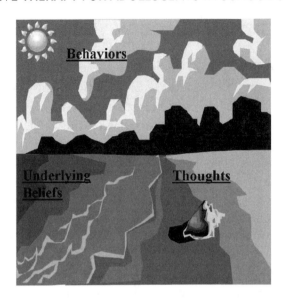

FIGURE 3.17. Air, land, water analogy.

CLINICIAN: Exactly! And that parallels the process people go through as they change. Changing your behavior over the course of a few days or weeks, like not avoiding stressful situations, will help to change your thinking. Can you imagine that?

ANJANAE: I guess. I mean, it's not like it's going to happen instantly. I can't just suddenly decide to think differently. But I guess it makes sense that after I try doing things differently for a while, I might start to think differently.

CLINICIAN: That's great, Anjanae. I'm so impressed by how open you are to thinking about these things. You really seem to get it! So let's keep going with this idea. At the beginning of the summer, even when it's been hot for a couple of weeks, what does water in the ocean feel like?

ANJANAE: Cold! I went to the beach last year in the beginning of June, and I couldn't stand going in the water. I was really hot, but the water was icy.

CLINICIAN: Right. But what if you had gone at the end of August? What do you think it would have felt like then?

ANJANAE: The water's always warm by the end of the summer. It is the only time I will swim.

CLINICIAN: Exactly. It takes a summer full of hot days to change the ocean water. By the end of the summer, the ocean has been heated up by all of the warm air and the warm ground that is near it. The same kind of thing is happening with you, Anjanae. It will take time, but you've been working so hard at changing your behavior patterns (like the air temperature) and your thinking patterns (like the ground temperature), and if you continue to do so it will change your underlying beliefs (like the ocean temperature).

This may be difficult for younger or lower functioning students to grasp, and you may want to use this analogy only with students whose treatment plans are anchored to their underlying beliefs. We have found that this analogy can make these ideas more concrete for students so that the cognitive model of change is a little easier for them to understand.

THE DOWNWARD ARROW

The main technique we recommend to identify underlying beliefs is the **downward arrow** (Burns, 1980). This technique was specifically designed to give the clinician and student a better understanding of the underlying core beliefs that are playing an active role in the student's difficulties. With students whose treatment plans are anchored to underlying beliefs, you will use the downward arrow to understand and show students how their underlying beliefs are related to their problems. However, it can also be used with students who have their treatment plans anchored to behavior and thought patterns. The downward arrow can help you to understand the underlying beliefs of these students and to form a solid cognitive conceptualization of them, even if they are not engaged in working on that deeper level.

> The downward arrow helps students to delve into the meaning of automatic thoughts, looking for underlying beliefs.

The downward arrow technique focuses on discovering with the student, "What does that [automatic thought] mean about you?" It is based on the understanding that students' automatic thoughts are a reflection of their beliefs about themselves and the world. In session, when a student's thought is a reflection of underlying negative beliefs, you will often see the student experience a negative emotion. When these beliefs are stirred up, or activated, she will experience feelings like sadness, anger, shame, or psychological pain. You will probably be able to read these feelings from the student's facial expression, body language, and other nonverbal cues. You will also notice that students will find it difficult to change these negative thoughts because such thoughts are closely tied to their underlying beliefs. These beliefs are the basis of their view of themselves and/or the world as well as the deep foundation for how they have been thinking for a long time.

This being said, underlying beliefs are often easier to modify in adolescents than they are in adults because they are more malleable, and in most cases, still developing and changing. Due to the foundational, developing nature of underlying beliefs in high school students, some of the most important and influential work can be done when examining and challenging their beliefs about themselves and the world. To identify underlying beliefs, begin by exploring with students what their automatic thoughts mean about them. This process cannot be forced and should only be carried out while the student is able to honestly delve into foundational and often embarrassing beliefs with the clinician. The following conversation shows the downward arrow being applied with Michele and provides an example of when it should be stopped or continued.

CLINICIAN: You said just now—"He is disgusted by me"—what else went through your mind when you thought that?

MICHELE: That I'm a fat pig.

CLINICIAN: And what does that mean about you?

MICHELE: He won't want to be with me.

CLINICIAN: So if he doesn't want to be with you, then what would that mean about you?

MICHELE: What the hell do you think? Are you stupid? It just sucks and I'm sick of it.

At this point, the clinician will need to be mindful of the student's feelings of safety and frustration, and should consider whether or not to continue with the downward arrow. Particularly for students with a history of sexual trauma or other situations where control has been taken from them, it is important to be aware of how invasive this technique can feel. In this situation, when Michele becomes resistant, we would recommend that the clinician address her automatic thoughts about the process in the session and/or explain that he wants to be mindful of her feelings and ask if she would prefer that he stop asking questions about this during that day's session. Alternatively, if Michele had not become resistant, the session might have gone as follows.

CLINICIAN: You said just now—"He is disgusted by me"—what else went through your mind when you thought that?

MICHELE: That I'm a fat pig.

CLINICIAN: And what does that mean about you?

MICHELE: He won't want to be with me.

CLINICIAN: So if he doesn't want to be with you, then what would that mean about you?

MICHELE: It's just a sign of how disgusting I am—that no one will ever want to be with me.

CLINICIAN: And if no one will ever want to be with you, then what would that say about you?

MICHELE: That I'm unlovable.

CLINICIAN: I can imagine how painful that must be to think. Painful beyond what the word even captures. . . I wonder if that belief about being unlovable might be at the core of some of your other beliefs.

The clinician should then continue to empathically reflect on how difficult her belief that she is unlovable is to have, while also exploring how that belief relates to her past and present behaviors and thoughts.

CHALLENGING AND CHANGING UNDERLYING BELIEFS

Challenging underlying beliefs can be done indirectly by helping the student change his behaviors and thinking patterns as described in this chapter and in Chapter 4. However, challenging underlying beliefs can also be done directly by applying guided discovery, checking the evidence, and other cognitive techniques. These techniques can be very effective, and for students who have their treatment anchored to underlying beliefs, you can help them make changes to their core view of themselves that can significantly improve their lives.

When directly challenging underlying beliefs, timing is important. In an ideal situation, you would *identify* underlying beliefs early in the session, and then *evaluate* underlying beliefs near the middle of the session. Challenging underlying beliefs in the middle of the session gives the student time to cope with the emotional effects of looking at the negative aspects of herself and so that she is able to leave the session feeling stable. Contrary to counseling provided in an outpatient setting, students usually have to return to class after a session, and they will need to be in an emotional state to do so. In light of this, you will want to make sure that the student is equipped with coping skills to handle the emotional distress that may accompany looking at and changing some of her underlying beliefs. If a student is in crisis, you would focus on coping skills and refrain from delving deeper into the underlying beliefs that relate to the crisis. In short, a student should never leave your office in tears or upset after uncovering underlying beliefs. If a student is in distress toward the end of the session, you may need to extend the session and/or focus on coping skills. Ideally, sessions that target underlying beliefs will follow a pattern similar to that in Figure 3.18.

Similarly, be mindful of the course of the school year when targeting underlying beliefs. Immediately prior to a long school break (summer vacation, spring break, etc.) is clinically

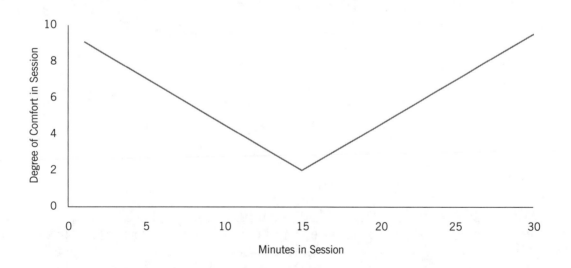

FIGURE 3.18. Discomfort and depth in session.

not a good time to begin challenging core beliefs, because you may not have enough time to support the student in digesting information and integrating new, more adaptive core beliefs. As with the session pattern diagram shown in Figure 3.18, counseling should be most emotionally taxing during middle sessions. A more comprehensive description of the counseling process as it takes place over the months of your work with the student will be provided in Chapter 5. Early sessions will focus on problem solving and changing behavior and thinking patterns; middle sessions will target the most difficult to change aspects of the student that are interfering with her meeting her counseling goals; and later sessions should focus on strengthening coping skills and relapse prevention. This pattern is depicted in the graph shown in Figure 3.19.

In reviewing the last narrative with Michele and her clinician, can you see where she may benefit from challenging her underlying belief of being unlovable (depending on where she is in the session and in the school year, of course)? One way to explore and then evaluate her belief would be to create a list of what would make someone lovable or unlovable. This list should not be about what would make *her* lovable or unlovable, as this may initially be too close to home. Instead, you would make a list with her about what would make *people in general* lovable or unlovable. The following session presents a narrative for how this approach could play out.

CLINICIAN: I'm really glad to see you again, Michele. What stood out for you the most about our last session?

MICHELE: Well, I remember that I cried through a lot of it, and we talked about my beliefs about being unlovable.

CLINICIAN: Right. I could see how hard it was for you, and I also remember the admirable and brave way you were openly discussing your beliefs with me.

MICHELE: Thanks.

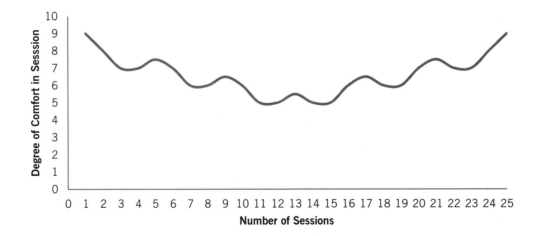

FIGURE 3.19. Distress and depth across sessions.

CLINICIAN: If it is OK with you, I would like to spend some time today thinking about what makes other people lovable. Can we spend today discussing that?

MICHELE: OK.

[Discussing what makes someone unlovable would only take place if Michele was not experiencing significant difficulties and was emotionally ready to do so. The following takes place after the clinician has made sure that this is the case.]

CLINICIAN: Let's write together some of the things that make someone lovable or unlovable.

MICHELE: OK.

The clinician and Michele would then brainstorm a list of everything that Michele believes makes someone worthy of being loved. After the list is created, Michele and her clinician may evaluate it by asking some of the following questions.

- Are the things on the "lovable list" really requirements for being loved?
- Are the things on the "unlovable list" really things that would make someone utterly unlovable?
- Is anyone really unlovable?

After evaluating the lists, Michele and her clinician would also consider how many of the lovable criteria items Michele actually meets (which would be many or most of them). If a student states that she does not meet the criteria for being lovable or capable, the clinician will then use guided discovery to help the student understand how she does meet the criteria, how the student can meet the criteria, or why the criteria should be changed. Students may have different criteria for other people than they have for themselves, often because they are harsher with themselves than with others. With continued guided discovery, the clinician can help students understand that the criteria they have for others should be the same criteria they have for themselves.

Students who were exposed to traumatic experience, grew up in chaotic homes, or live in a dangerous neighborhood may have a view of the world as dangerous that persists even when they are around "safe" people or situations. These views of the world can be very problematic, because they can interfere with the student trusting people or letting their guard down when they should. For instance, Michele, who was exposed to sexual abuse at an early age, may have a view of all men as dangerous and as only interested in her for sex. This view, if left unexamined, would interfere with her ability to develop relationships with males who do care about her.

Michele's core belief that men are dangerous, or in her words, that "boys are only interested in one thing," results in her intermediate belief that "The only way to get what I want from males [attention, caring, etc.] is to give them what they want [sex]." This belief has resulted in a pattern of behavior in which Michele engages in sexual relations with boys in hopes that they will "love" her. However, she is continually let down when she is viewed only as a sexual target as a result of her behavior patterns. To help Michele evaluate this intermediate belief and this behavior pattern, the clinician could help her identify the two and collaboratively explore how they have worked for her in the past. The clinician and Michele could then consider alternative behaviors. The following narrative is an example of how this conversation might go.

CLINICIAN: You've really been doing a great job of openly discussing your beliefs and the kind of things you have been doing. I really appreciate your bravery in doing this, and I was hoping we could take a look at what you have been doing and at some alternative ways of doing things.

MICHELE: OK.

CLINICIAN: So let's look at what happened with you and Steve.

MICHELE: Uh, do we have to?

CLINICIAN: Of course not, and it is your decision. I only chose what happened with Steve because it is recent, and it seemed similar to what happened with a couple of the other guys you've talked about. But again, we can pick someone else, or not do this activity at all.

MICHELE: OK . . . we can talk about what happened with Steve.

[Note: If Michele had decided not to talk about the situation with Steve, the clinician could explore Michele's reasons for not wanting to talk about him. Does she think that she will be judged by the clinician? Is she telling herself that her behavior was too shameful to talk about? Does she think that her sexual behavior is not an important topic in counseling? Understanding Michele's hesitation can provide important information for the clinician about Michele's thoughts and beliefs.]

CLINICIAN: How will I know if you want to stop the activity or if I am going too fast or too slow?

MICHELE: I'll tell you.

CLINICIAN: Good. You're really good at keeping me posted on what is going on with you as we work together. So, what were your initial thoughts when you considered sleeping with Steve?

MICHELE: I remember thinking that he will leave me if I don't.

CLINICIAN: Good job identifying the thought. And let's take a look at that. You did decide to sleep with him . . . and what ended up happening?

MICHELE: He dumped me. He's such a jerk.

CLINICIAN: I know how hard this is for you, Michele. . . . You're doing a great job with this. Let's look at your thinking.

MICHELE: Well, I was right! He actually really is a jerk! I was pretty stupid for thinking that he would stay with me if I slept with him.

CLINICIAN: So, it seems like your thinking that sleeping with Steve would keep him around was not so accurate.

MICHELE: Yeah.

CLINICIAN: Do you think that there are some guys who would stay with you, even if you don't sleep with them?

MICHELE: Not Steve, or any of the other guys I dated!

CLINICIAN: Well, you may be on to something. What did your relationship with Steve and with the other guys you have dated have in common?

MICHELE: They all liked me at first, and then they took off. I must really be unlovable.

CLINICIAN: I'm not so sure we know that they took off because you're "unlovable." What do you remember about how each of these relationships started off?

MICHELE: I flirted with them, and then we hooked up, and the minute I sleep with them, they take off!

Before you continue reading, take a moment to write down how you would make sense of what Michele is saying and how you would respond.

What is the belief that is driving Michele's pattern of behavior?

_____

_____

_____

How could you help Michele to evaluate that belief?

_____

_____

_____

Did you identify Michele's belief that the only way she can catch and maintain a boy's interest in her is through sex?

[Here is one way that the clinician could help Michele to test that belief. The clinician reviews with Michele the list of criteria for being lovable, and the ways in which she meets those criteria.]

MICHELE: Yeah, I guess I do see that I have a lot of things that make me lovable. Still, none of them seem to see it.

CLINICIAN: Well, now let's spend some time thinking about that. We've already talked a little bit about how these relationships start and the pattern that plays out. What do you remember about that?

MICHELE: It usually starts with flirting—me or them—and then we end up getting together. There's usually sex pretty soon after that, and then the guy is gone. They're with me, but they never see all this supposedly "lovable" stuff about me.

CLINICIAN: Well, let's take some guesses about how that happens. Imagine that when someone starts to get to know you, they're looking at you through a pair of sunglasses. When the relationship starts off with sex, the sunglasses that he picks up are the "sex" sunglasses, so that's the lens he sees you through. Now imagine a different guy who gets to know you without the relationship starting off sexually. Maybe you start as friends, or helping each other with homework, or something else that doesn't have anything related to sex. What kind of sunglasses would he see you through?

MICHELE: I don't know—I guess it would depend. He could see me through a "friend" lens, or a "smart" lens, or something like that.

CLINICIAN: Good! So, which lens is going to help this guy see all of the parts that make you lovable?

MICHELE: Maybe the "friend" or "smart" lenses, but does that mean that the only way to keep a good guy is to never have sex with him, even if we date into college and then decide to have sex? Because that's not what I want!

CLINICIAN: Great question! Let's look at that. If a boy sees you through the "friend" lens, and as you described, you both wait till college to have sex, would that take away all the things he already liked about you?

MICHELE: Maybe not. I don't know. I know that you're trying to say that he'd still like all those other things, and just get to see more of who I am, but I'm not sure that's true.

CLINICIAN: I can understand why you're not so sure. I wonder if we could try testing it out . . . I know you've been spending time with James lately. Could we think of a way to try testing out the idea that waiting will lead to him leaving you?

In this narrative, the clinician is careful to not shame Michele. Instead, the clinician helps her consider other ways that she can build a relationship and test her belief that the only way to keep a boy interested in her is to sleep with him. The clinician makes references to the "lens" boys might use to see her, using that analogy to talk about the thoughts boys might have about her. Exploring and changing her behavior patterns will help Michele change underlying beliefs about herself and boys as well as help her develop a safe pattern of behaving. If the clinician were to shame her or demand that she never sleep with boys, he would be replaying the process of taking control away from her and subsequently reinforcing her belief that she is unlovable and out of control. Clinicians who use shame or lecturing as an approach are likely to find that students stop coming to counseling or refrain from discussing core problematic beliefs, thoughts, and behavior patterns.

SUPPORTING EVIDENCE

Although the effectiveness of CT has been widely studied and supported, there is surprisingly little research on the ways in which specific techniques help to create change. However, there is a great deal of evidence that clients' thoughts are related to their disorders, including depression (Gotlib & Joormann, 2010; Romens, Abramson & Alloy, 2009), anxiety (Cisler & Koster, 2010; Clerkin & Teachman, 2010), substance abuse (Lee, Pohlman, Baker, Ferris, & Kay-Lambkin, 2010), psychosis (Mawson, Cohen & Berry, 2010), posttraumatic stress disorder (Bennett & Wells, 2010; Cromer & Smyth, 2010), and other disorders. Techniques such as thought records, the Three C's, the downward arrow, and others are the vehicles through which clients identify, evaluate, and modify their thoughts and in turn make changes in their symptoms.

A few studies have looked at cognitive changes (using the techniques in this chapter) and how those changes lead to changes in symptoms. A study by DeRubeis and Feeley (1990) found that cognitive changes predicted changes in clients' symptoms. Segal, Gemar, and Williams (1999) found that CT led to changes in schema (or core beliefs), while pharmacotherapy (medication) did not, showing that CT is helping clients make changes to their belief systems. Later, Segal and colleagues (2006) showed that clients who had received CT for depression were less likely to have a strong reaction to situations that would cause a sad mood than clients who had received medication for their depression, and that clients who reacted strongly (like those who did not receive CT) were more likely to have a relapse and become depressed again. Clients who reported that their mood changed significantly during a CT session also reported that they had had a meaningful cognitive change during the session (Persons & Burns, 1985), which provided support for the relationship between cognitive changes and changes in emotion. Finally, clients who were more skilled at filling out a thought record were significantly less depressed even 6 months after group CBT for depression than the clients who struggled with the thought record (Neimeyer & Feixas, 1990).

SUMMARY

There are many CT techniques that can be used when problem solving is not enough. The techniques in this chapter—thought bubbles, guided discovery, the Three C's, coping cards, replacement thoughts, thought records, the reverse role play, and the downward arrow can be applied in a variety of ways to address the unique problems that your students face. The techniques can be implemented in ways that tap the creativity and strengths that you and your students bring to each session, so that sessions are individually tailored and engaging. Be aware when choosing techniques of how they address the problems and treatment anchors that are interfering with your students reaching their goals.

In using these cognitive techniques, we invite you to see yourself as a warm and caring coach who teaches athletes techniques for winning games. Like the coach, you will explain how the student can use and apply techniques step by step, go through them with the student in session, and then encourage the student to practice and use the techniques outside of therapy. Also like a coach, you should expect the student to practice the techniques between sessions and then report back in the next session about how she is doing and what questions she has. When the student sees you as a caring coach who expects her to practice outside of session, it will help her to maximize the impact of each session and expand her learning to the real world problems she faces now and in the future.

CHAPTER 4

Behavioral Techniques

Behavioral techniques are an important complement to the cognitive techniques we have discussed so far. In fact, some of your most fruitful work will be done by focusing on behaviors, and some of these behavioral techniques may already be familiar to you. Behaviors are often the first place in which school systems intervene with adolescents. Teachers, principals and vice principals, lunch supervision staff, and other school staff often intervene with students' problematic behavior because it is what they see disrupting their class, creating problems in the cafeteria, and resulting in fights in the hallway. For example, rewarding good behavior and taking away privileges for bad behavior are behavioral strategies used by school staff for discipline and behavior management. However, the behavioral techniques we present here may focus on different behaviors than those the other school staff are targeting or they may target the behaviors in a different way. When done well, school staff members who intervene at a behavioral level are usually fairly effective at creating change in the short term (making the problem behavior go away for now). However, you as the cognitive clinician will be focused on both the short- and long-term effect of interventions on the student and school, making you responsible for helping students change their behavior both in the moment and in the future. This focus, combined with CT skills, will enable you to understand why interventions work and fail, helping both the student and the school. Rather than being a disciplinarian (which may be the role of those other staff), you will work as a team with your students to make changes; this approach requires a different way of working with behavior.

> **Behavioral techniques in CT target not only *behavior* change, but also a resulting change in *thoughts*.**

To return to the general cognitive model that we presented in the beginning of the book, a person's thoughts, feelings, and behavior are all related to and influence each other. In Chapter 3, we presented the cognitive triangle (Clarke et al., 1990). Most of this book has focused on the "thoughts" angle of this triangle, where you directly help students to work with their thinking to make changes in how they feel and act. Coming from a different angle, behavioral strategies help students to make changes in the way they behave, which indirectly leads to changes in how they think and feel. Cognitive and behavioral strategies can be used together to help students to make changes from multiple "angles." (See Figure 4.1.)

Behavioral strategies are often planned in session with students, and students then practice the behavioral strategies outside of the session. You and the student will work together in the session to identify a behavior that would be a good target for change, and then make a detailed plan about exactly when, where, and how to try to apply the behavioral strategy. The actual application of the strategy can happen anywhere—in the classroom, the lunchroom, out in the community, or at home. When the student returns to your office for the next session, the two of you will process what went well, what was harder than antici-pated, and how the student can take what she learned and apply it in a new situation. These behavioral strategies can build on each other to ultimately make meaningful change, just as cognitive strategies build on each other. Whether your counseling with the student is anchored to change in thinking or behavior patterns or anchored to deeper level change in core beliefs, behavioral strategies can be a powerful way to test out beliefs and learn from evidence, rather than learning based on assumptions.

This description of behavioral strategies may sound vague, because the strategies will vary a great deal depending on the student's presenting problem, existing skills, the degree to which the family is able to participate, whether counseling is anchored to thinking and behavior patterns or core beliefs, and other factors. The common factor among these behav-ioral strategies is that you and the student will work together to make a systematic plan for specific things the student will do based on the issues you are working on together and your case conceptualization. After the student tries to follow the plan, you will help him to process how the plan unfolded; how the student felt before, during and after the plan; and what he can learn from the process.

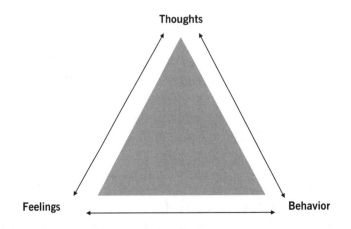

FIGURE 4.1. A different view of the cognitive model (based on Clarke et al., 1990).

In the following section, we will present the behavioral strategies that we have found to be most useful in a school counseling setting. These include behavioral experiments, behavioral activation, safety plans, hope kits, replacement behaviors, exposures, progressive relaxation, and meditation. Although you can certainly use other behavioral strategies, these form the basis of much of the CT work done in schools.

BEHAVIORAL EXPERIMENTS

Behavioral experiments (Beck, 1995) are very closely related to cognitive interventions. When beliefs are identified that may be unrealistic, one way of challenging those beliefs is to evaluate their accuracy by setting up a situation that tests the student's expectations. Often, behavioral experiments are used when a student assumes that something negative will happen in a certain situation, even though he cannot know for sure that anything bad will happen. For example, David told his clinician that he believes that if he were to ever admit to anyone that he was gay, he would be rejected and ridiculed. He firmly believes this to be fact. Therefore, he has never admitted to anyone except his best friend

> Remember to plan for a wide range of possible outcomes. What if things go well? What if the worst-case scenario takes place? What about mixed results?

(who originally brought him to the clinician's office) that he is gay. His best friend was supportive when he told her, but he still believes that no one but she would accept him, and therefore he keeps his sexuality a secret. This silence has resulted in David having very few friends, and he feels very alone and isolated. In a behavioral experiment, David and his clinician would set up a situation in which they could evaluate his intermediate belief that if he told anyone that he is gay, then they would reject him. This experiment would take careful planning, because the clinician would want to set up the situation so that David had the maximum chance for success—in other words, the maximum chance that he would *not* be rejected. They would work together to make a plan, including ideas about:

- *Whom to tell:* Who might be most likely to be open to his sexuality? Who would respect his privacy and not repeat the information?
- *What to say:* How much information does David want to share? What is he comfortable saying, and what kind of language does he want to use? Is there anything David wants to plan to *not* share in this conversation?
- *When to have the conversation:* What would create good timing or bad timing? When can he plan to have the conversation? What would be a sign that he should wait for a better time?
- *Where:* Is there a setting where he can have the conversation in privacy? Where would he feel comfortable?
- *How:* How does David want to share the information? How can he say it in a way that makes it most likely that the other person will be understanding and accepting?

Once David and his clinician have thought through a plan, they will do role plays to practice how David might handle some of the different ways that the conversation might go. A key piece of this planning is to think through *all* of the possible outcomes. Although David and his clinician will have done all that they can to make sure that the conversation goes well, they cannot control the listener's response. In other words, they will plan for the best and prepare for the worst. These preparations will include ways to handle any outcome during the conversation (What will David say if he gets a negative reaction? How will he respond to a positive reaction? How will he end the conversation?), as well as thoughts that he can say to himself during and after the conversation ("This person is reacting badly, but that is more about him being closed-minded than about something being wrong with me"; "No matter how this turns out, I am proud of myself for trying"; "I am strong enough to handle anything that happens here"; "I feel freer just telling someone, no matter how that person reacts.").

After planning this conversation in the clinician's office, David would put his plan into action. After the conversation takes place, he would come back to his clinician to talk about how the plan worked out. Regardless of the outcome, there is something to be learned. If David did not go forward with the plan, he and his clinician can talk about what got in the way. What was David saying to himself that kept him from trying the plan? What went wrong? If he did go forward with the plan and the conversation went well, what does that tell him about his intermediate belief that he will be rejected by anyone he tells that he is gay? If the conversation went poorly, what did he learn about his ability to cope with his feared outcome? Is there something he could do differently next time? Was he more able to handle disappointment than he thought he would be?

Just as in the rest of life, behavioral interventions do not always go the way we plan or hope. However, the key is knowing that there is some insight to be gained, no matter how the experiment turns out. If the experiment goes well, then the student's negative belief can be undermined or shifted in a more helpful and healthy direction. If it does not go well, the clinician and student have planned enough in advance that they can learn from the experience and apply that knowledge when they try again. In working with students in situations similar to David's, we have found that they were frequently able to see that they can handle setbacks and were proud that they tried something difficult. After the situation is discussed, the clinician and student then take what they learned and plan a new behavioral experiment.

Think of a student you are working with now or have worked with in the past. What was an assumption that the student made and assumed was true, without testing out the facts? How did that assumption dictate how the student handled other situations? How could you set up a behavioral experiment to test out the assumption? Remember to plan for the experiment to go well *or* not so well!

_____

_____

_____

_____

_____

_____

_____

_____

_____

_____

_____

BEHAVIORAL ACTIVATION

Behavioral activation (Beck, 1995) is a strategy used most often with students who are depressed. When students become depressed, they usually do fewer and fewer fun activities. A cycle then begins: As the student does fewer activities for fun, the subsequent reduction of pleasure in her life leads to more depression, which then leaves the student even less motivated to have fun, and so on. This same cycle also reduces the student's social interactions and social support. The less the student does, the less she interacts with others, and that social isolation leads to more depression and less motivation to be active. In order to reverse this cycle, you can work with your student to plan pleasurable activities. The activities that are planned should be ones in which the student already feels some sense of mastery. Over time, choosing activities that help the student increase her sense of mastery will also help to reduce thoughts and feelings related to depression. For example, slowly building a sense of competence in social situations, sports, hobbies, and other enjoyable activities will increase the time that the student spends in those activities, as well as her sense of being skilled in these areas.

The first step in this process is to get a sense of how much fun and pleasure the student already has in her life. For example, you may ask Michele to write down each time she does something during the week that is fun or makes her feel happy. This would give you and Michele a starting place for knowing what makes Michele happy now. Together, you can then schedule specific times for Michele to enjoy those pursuits, so that they happen more often during the week. Michele may also make a list of activities that would be pleasurable for her. This list should include activities that are accessible to her with the resources she has. For example, going for a swim may be something Michele loves to do, but it is only appropriate for the list if Michele has access to a pool. Spending a weekend in New York City may not be accessible for most people, but if Michele has family there whom she could visit and a way to get there for the weekend, it may be an appropriate activity for her list. If Michele has trouble thinking of activities that would be fun, you and she could refer to the list of pleasant activities in Appendix 4.1 for ideas. The two of you should also consider whether there are any negatives that are likely to be associated with the fun activity. For example, given the beliefs that Michele has about boys and sex, planning an intimate moment with a boy would not be a good choice for her. Even if it would cause happiness in the moment, she may ultimately pay a price emotionally for it.

Whether the activities chosen are current activities that Michele is planning to do more often, or new activities she is adding to her week, a key step is planning specifically when and how she will participate in them. For example, planning to spend a weekend in New York is not enough for a student who is depressed, even if she has access to a way to make the trip. Without additional planning, Michele is not likely to actually go to New York. Depressed students often have a very hard time getting started on an activity (particularly a big event like a trip), which is why these activities decrease with depression. However, if you and Michele make a step-by-step plan, the chances that Michele will follow through are increased. The planning may look similar to the planning above in the behavioral experiment.

- *What to do:* Specifically, what would be a fun activity for Michele? What are all of the steps involved in participating in the activity?
- *How:* How will Michele participate in the activity? Does she have the resources she needs? What steps does she need to take to make the activity possible?
- *Who:* Whom will Michele include in the activity? If someone else is involved, is it someone who will create a barrier (e.g., say that he or she can't participate) or will he or she be likely to support Michele's plans?
- *Where:* Where is the best place for Michele to do the activity she is planning?
- *When:* When exactly will Michele do the activity? On which day and at what time will she do it? What could get in the way of her being able to do it at that time?

You and Michele should plan for anything that might derail her plans. For example, you could role-play Michele asking her relatives if she can visit them in New York, and then she may even call them from your office to actually ask them. You may also think together of any barriers that may keep her from participating in the enjoyable activities and then plan to sidestep the barriers. Michele may say that she cannot go swimming at the YMCA, even though she has a membership, because she does not have a bathing suit. You can then problem-solve about ways that Michele can have something to wear to swim. When all of the planning is complete, the plan should be written down so that Michele has all of the details easily accessible.

After making a specific written plan for fun activities during the week, Michele would put her plan into action. In the next session, she would discuss with you how the plan worked. As with a behavioral experiment, there is something to be learned regardless of the outcome. If Michele did not go forward with the plan, you can think together about what got in the way. If things go well, then you and she will process how she felt before, during, and after the activity. It will be particularly important to explore with Michele *how changing her behavior changed her mood, and how those changes might impact her beliefs.* For example, if enjoys the trip to New York to visit her family, her positive interactions with the people there might be evidence for her that she has value beyond what she can offer sexually. If Michele's mood lightens at all during her trip, her belief that food, sex, and cutting herself are the only ways she can change or improve her mood would also be evaluated. As Michele continues to build more enjoyable activities into her week, the increased moments of happiness, activity, and social interaction will also support the work she is doing in session with you to help decrease her depression.

SCHOOL-BASED COGNITIVE THERAPY FOR SUICIDAL THOUGHTS

Adolescence is known to be a high-risk time for the emergence of suicidal thinking and behavior. In 2006, suicide was the third leading cause of death for 10- to 14-year-olds and 15- to 19-year-olds in the United States (Centers for Disease Control and Prevention, 2006). The likelihood that clinicians working with adolescents in school settings will see this issue is therefore very high. Depending on the laws and policies in your setting, students who are at risk for causing serious harm to themselves (or others) may need a more intensive level of care than is provided in a typical school setting. Therefore, referrals should be facilitated for students whose safety is in question. For students whose thoughts are related to suicide but who are still appropriate candidates for services offered in your setting, the use of cognitive strategies presented in the previous chapter (which are very highly recommended for students with suicidal thinking), plus the following specific behavioral strategies, may be appropriate.

> **Remember to assess whether students need a higher level of care than you can provide in a school and to follow all school policies and local laws.**

Your work in the school setting creates an opportunity for collaboration with important others in a student's life. Schools are a unique environment where peers and teachers can have a powerful impact on the student. One way in which you can be particularly effective is by educating other school staff about warning signs for suicide. Taking a two-pronged approach is often effective: offer information to all school staff during an inservice or other opportunity, and then speak directly with any staff whom at-risk students have identified as a resource. Again, remember to check the privacy laws in your state and the policies in your school district before sharing this information, because some states and districts may require the student's explicit permission before you can do so.

Another important step to take is to communicate to students and staff that telling you that a friend or student is suicidal is *not* betraying the student's trust. Teachers, peers, and others often feel trapped when a student confides in them that he or she is thinking about suicide, under the condition of keeping that fact a secret. Communicate to peers and teachers that keeping secrets about suicide is a bigger betrayal of the student than sharing the secret. Peers, in particular, will often relate to the idea that it is better to have a friend alive and angry that you shared a secret, than dead with their secret kept.

Hope Kit

Developing a **hope kit** is a behavioral strategy that is often used when students are experiencing suicidal thoughts, although hope kits can also be powerful for students who are experiencing less than suicidal levels of distress (Wenzel, Brown, & Beck, 2009). Students can develop a hope kit on their own or with help from you. Most commonly, a hope kit is an actual box, decorated by the student and filled with items that help the student to feel inspired, optimistic, or hopeful about the future. A key item for the student to include in a hope kit is a list of **reasons for living** (see Appendix 4.2 at the end of the book) and a list of **pros and cons for living** (see Appendix 4.3 at the end of the book). These lists should be developed during a session so that the student has support in thinking through the reasons that inspire them to stay alive, the pros and cons of doing so, and evaluating the power of the reasons on the lists. The ideas should be primarily generated by the student so that they resonate with him or her and carry enough emotional weight to be convincing, even in a moment of crisis. However, you can be very helpful in guiding the student toward items for the list.

In addition to a list of reasons for living, and a list of pros and cons for living, the student may include anything else in the box that inspires hope for him or her. Many students have included pictures, poetry, letters, prayer cards, coping cards, Bible verses, or other items that help them to stay anchored in the positive. A particularly important role for you as the counselor is to help the student evaluate these choices. For example, Anjanae may suggest putting a sonogram picture in her hope kit. If the picture leaves her consistently feeling inspired and optimistic, then the picture would be a good choice for the hope kit. If, however, she sometimes becomes overwhelmed or distressed in thinking about how the baby would affect on her life, then the picture would not be a good choice. Items that are included should provide consistent positive feelings and thoughts.

The hope kit can be built into a plan as part of the student's coping strategies. It can also stand as a behavioral strategy in its own right, providing a source of positive thought and emotion for a student who needs an anchor in those things. When the student realizes that he or she is thinking distressing thoughts or feeling down, going through the hope kit can be very helpful. Sharing the hope kit with a trusted friend or family member can also be an effective way of increasing support for the student.

REPLACEMENT BEHAVIORS

Adolescents sometimes have specific behaviors that are problematic, particularly in a school setting. For example, a student may wander the halls or classroom, boss around less popular students, and yell out inappropriate answers in class. These kinds of behavior issues are often managed by teachers and other disciplinary staff. However, the behaviors can become therapy issues when the student can identify the behavior as a personal problem, or when the behavior is interfering with the student achieving what she wants in life. These behaviors should be identified as part of the anchor plan for treatment, because of that interference. The behavior may be costing a student a spot on the honor roll or a sports team, or it may be landing the student in detention or suspension. When a student has a specific behavior that is problematic, developing a **replacement behavior** can help to reduce or end the problem behavior (Baer et al., 1968, 1987; O'Neill, Horner, Alpin, Sprague, Storey, & Newton, 1997). However, we strongly recommend that cognitive work be done along with planning a replacement behavior.

Replacement behaviors work best in conjunction with cognitive work around the reasons that the original behavior exists, and cognitive work may be necessary before the student recognizes that the problem behavior is actually causing a problem for her. The first step in replacing a problem behavior is working collaboratively with the student, perhaps through guided discovery, to identify the goal of the behavior. What is the student trying to achieve with the behavior? What need does it meet? Once the real goal of the behavior is identified, the student and clinician can work to find a different behavior that provides a more appropriate way to meet the need while making the problem behavior (Crone & Horner, 2003):

- *Irrelevant* (the problem behavior now has no purpose or does not work).
- *Inefficient* (the problem behavior does not work as well as a more appropriate behavior).
- *Ineffective* (the problem behavior no longer achieves the desired goal).

Michele has talked about cutting herself as a way to release stress, upset, and other negative emotions when she starts to feel overwhelmed by them. If we were to help her replace her cutting behavior with journaling, for example, the cutting would become *irrelevant*. The cutting would no longer serve the purpose of releasing negative emotions, because she would be able to take care of those emotions by writing in her journal as soon as she started to recognize those emotions. Anjanae described her sexual relationship with her boyfriend as the only thing she has been doing "just for myself," and that sexual activity has led to an unplanned pregnancy. If she were to replace unprotected sex with other, less risky self-care activities (like a bubble bath, a long walk outside, reading a book for fun), she may come to see unprotected sex as an *inefficient* way of making herself feel better and of taking care of herself. The less risky behaviors can help her feel just as happy and fulfilled, without the anxiety and stress related to unprotected sex. For David, feeling "different" because he is gay has led him to pull away from his friends. However, this approach, instead of helping David to feel less different, makes him feel even less connected to others. If David were to work with his clinician to find a way to reach out to the people who value and care about him when he feels really down about himself, that would show that the withdrawal was really just an *ineffective* way of dealing with his feelings.

Table 4.1 provides examples of the ways in which student's needs can be met by appropriate or inappropriate behavior. Once the need and inappropriate behavior are identi-

TABLE 4.1. Needs, Unwanted Behavior, and Replacement Behavior

Need	Unwanted behavior	Replacement behavior
For attention	Yelling out "smart" answers in class.	Raises hand, responds to teacher's question, and is praised.
To feel in charge	Bossing students with less social power.	Acts as the leader of a group project.
To be active instead of sitting at the desk	Wandering around the classroom or halls.	Is responsible for delivering attendance sheets to office (with a time limit).

fied by the student and clinician, they can work together to brainstorm other behaviors that could meet the need in a more appropriate manner. The final step of this strategy involves increasing the desired behavior to meet the need, so that the inappropriate behavior becomes unnecessary and is ultimately replaced.

For example, Alfred's fighting has had a negative effect on his spot on the wrestling team and on his grades, and it has placed his chances for a scholarship at risk. For the first several sessions of therapy, Alfred denied that his fighting was a problem. Instead, he saw it as the only way to keep others from taking advantage of him. After you and he spend a number of sessions working on this underlying belief ("If I don't always strike first, I'll end up as a weak victim"), Alfred has started to consider the possibility that being aggressive is not always the best approach to a problem. Although it sometimes does seem to solve problems in a short-term sense while in the streets, the long-term consequences of being aggressive in school far outweigh the benefits. He may scare off someone who is bothering him, but he realizes that the person often returns with additional people to bother him again. He also worries about the example he is setting for his younger brother, and the effect that the fighting has had on his wrestling, grades, and future scholarships. Once Alfred recognizes that his fighting behavior is a problem for him while in school and that he would like to change it, you and he begin to work on a replacement behavior. Alfred was fighting to help himself feel powerful instead of vulnerable. Together, you consider other ways that Alfred can feel powerful, without the high costs of fighting. He brainstorms a list of possibilities, including:

- Yelling and threatening.
- Walking away.
- Cutting the other person down by saying mean things.
- Saving face by making a joke.
- Reporting the other student to school staff.

Reporting the other student to school staff is immediately crossed off the list, because Alfred knows that "snitching" would only make his peers look down on him and target him more. Yelling, threatening, and cutting the other person down are crossed off of the list because Alfred decides that those behaviors are likely to lead to fighting. Alfred decides that combining the last two options, walking away while saying something funny to save face, seems like his best choice. You and Alfred practice several role plays, where you discover that Alfred has a quick sense of humor that can de-escalate a difficult situation. His disarming jokes prevent him from feeling vulnerable, sidestep the fight, and may even get him some positive attention. You reinforce that he needs to pair his jokes with walking away, because remaining in the situation while making jokes could just make the problem worse. Alfred agrees to watch for a situation during the week in which he can try this new tactic for homework and report back in the next session. In planning for that next session, you remember to focus on how well the replacement behavior worked and how Alfred's experience relates to his thoughts and beliefs about striking first.

For some students, jokes may work in the opposite way, escalating a problem or a fight. "Jokes" that are actually sarcastic statements, jabs at the other person, or other destructive behavior can create a larger problem rather than easing the tension. Using gentle humor to decrease a problem is a difficult skill to build, as many therapists learn when they first try to use humor in therapy. Be careful when students plan to use humor to help resolve situations, making sure that the humor they use improves a situation rather than making it worse. Role plays can be a great way to check this, along with reviewing times in the past when the student used humor successfully (or not).

EXPOSURE

Students with anxiety can gain significant benefits from **exposure tasks** (Albano & Kendall, 2002; Kendall et al., 2005). Exposures are a behavioral intervention aimed at reversing some of the processes at work in anxiety. In an anxious situation, students will first experience automatic thoughts about their inability to handle a situation they perceive as threatening. Students with chronic anxiety, or anxiety that gets in their way, misperceive danger that is not really part of the situation or greatly underestimate their ability to handle it. It is human nature to avoid situations that are too dangerous to manage, so the student tries avoidance as a compensatory strategy. The avoidance prevents students from ever checking or correcting their negative, helpless automatic thoughts about the situation, so that the anxious automatic thoughts become more deeply rooted and the anxiety is reinforced in an ongoing cycle. (See Figure 4.2.)

In exposure tasks, you and the student first work to identify the student's automatic thoughts in anxious situations. The student then generates a **fear hierarchy** of situations that would make him or her progressively more nervous (Kendall et al., 2005). The hierarchy should begin with a situation that would make the student only mildly nervous, followed by a somewhat harder situation, all the way up to a very frightening situation. Each step on the hierarchy should be related to the same overall fear, building up from a small "dose" of the fear to a very large "dose." Anjanae and her clinician have been working on her fears about giving a presentation in front of her class. An example of the fear hierarchy they built together is found in Figure 4.3, and a blank worksheet for building a hierarchy can be found in Appendix 4.4 at the end of the book.

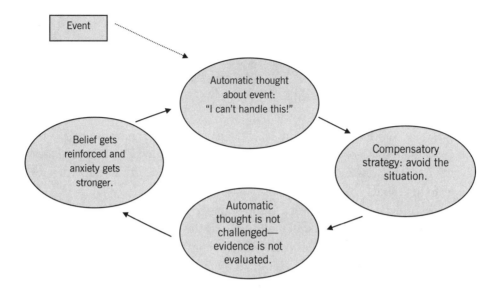

FIGURE 4.2. The avoidance–anxiety cycle.

Along with ranking situations in terms of how anxiety-provoking they would be, the clinician would teach Anjanae about SUDS (Subjective Units of Distress; Wolpe, 1969) ratings. In these ratings, a scale of 0–100 points indicates how much anxiety a situation causes. You may find it helpful to show students a ratings scale to describe SUDS; some students may then be able to use the rating scale without having a physical scale in front of them. For the students who want to use a written scale for ratings, an example of a scale is included in Appendix 4.5 at the end of the book.

Anjanae then prepares to face the first (lowest) anxiety-provoking situation. A first exposure should be in session with the clinician whenever possible, but over time, exposures will make great homework assignments, so that Anjanae can practice using her coping skills in real situations. She should start preparing by identifying her automatic thoughts about the first situation. As described in Chapter 3 on cognitive techniques, those thoughts are caught, checked, and changed, and Anjanae will develop coping thoughts to deal with her unhelpful or inaccurate thoughts. A coping card can be written out, or Anjanae can simply practice repeating the coping thoughts. Next, Anjanae and her clinician will practice any of the other cognitive or behavioral strategies that help her face the situation. Role-playing

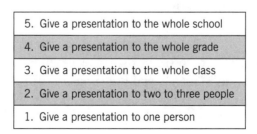

FIGURE 4.3. Sample fear hierarchy for Anjanae's fear of speaking in public.

ways for her to handle being in front of a person or people during a presentation, relaxation, and problem solving are particularly helpful. Just as in a behavioral experiment, remember to maximize the likelihood that Anjanae will be successful, but prepare for any potential problems.

A key factor for success is that she must stay in the situation until she has reached her goal, rather than avoiding the situation because of fear. For example, it is not enough for Anjanae to stand in front of the class for a moment and say three words if the goal was to read a paragraph to the class. Avoiding the situation by saying three words and then leaving the room will only reinforce her belief that she cannot handle this situation. Therefore, planning an exposure task that is a small, yet achievable, step forward is preferable to planning a larger step that may overwhelm the student. The clinician may be tempted to stop the exposure if Anjanae gets nervous in front of the group, but stopping at that point would really just reinforce her beliefs that she cannot handle presentations in front of groups. Building and practicing coping skills before the exposure to maximize the likelihood that the student can cope is also very important.

Facing the fear, rather than avoiding it, provides a student an opportunity to have a successful coping experience, which will both increase her sense of mastery and accomplishment and provide evidence against the automatic thoughts of being unable to handle the "dangerous" situation. Successes should be reinforced and celebrated. After the exposure task, process with the student what he liked about how he coped, what could be done differently next time, and anything else that he learned from the experience. The student can also use evidence from the exposure to see if the negative prediction he had was really accurate. On the basis of what you and the student learn from this successful coping experience, you can go on to plan an exposure to the next step in the hierarchy, eventually making it to the top step in the hierarchy. (See Figure 4.4.)

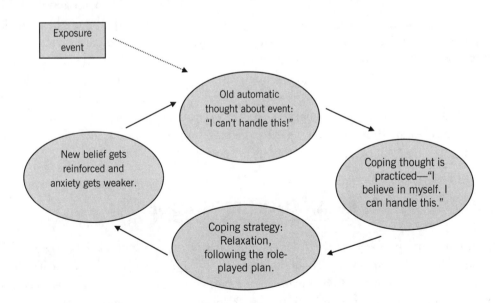

FIGURE 4.4. The exposure–anxiety reduction cycle.

To make the idea of exposure tasks more concrete, let's continue to follow Anjanae as she works her way through the fear hierarchy listed in Figure 4.3. She has already successfully accomplished the easiest step on her hierarchy—giving a presentation to one person. From that exposure, she learned that she was able to remember what she wanted to talk about (even though she predicted she would forget), that the listener did not make fun of her, and that she was able to answer a few easy questions at the end. She also learned that her hands sweated a lot during the presentation (which she had not expected). You and she already developed coping thoughts for the first exposure, including:

- "I'm smart, and this is a topic I know a lot about."
- "Even if I make a mistake, that will be OK, because everyone makes mistakes."

She decides to add a coping thought for the next exposure:

- "I did this once before, and it went better than I thought, so I will probably do well again."

She then role-plays her presentation to the larger group, with you and an additional staff member listening to her practice her speech and asking her questions. Anjanae also practices some deep breathing exercises she has learned from you (presented in the next section) so that she can stay relaxed. She decides that she will keep one tissue in each pocket to wipe her hands if they sweat. Finally, you and she agree that you will celebrate over ice cream if she successfully copes. Anjanae then presents her talk to three listeners, using her coping skills to successfully complete the exposure. After the exposure task, you spend time with Anjanae processing what you each have learned from the experience about the evidence for or against her fearful thoughts. A key question in processing the experience is to ask, "What does your success mean about you?" In challenging Anjanae's original fearful thought and beliefs by looking at her successful coping experience, you will be targeting some of the thoughts in the anchor plan for counseling. After processing what Anjanae liked about how she coped, what she would like to do differently the next time, and what she learned from the experience, you and she share ice cream from the cafeteria to celebrate (reinforce) how hard she worked on her thoughts and behavior. Then, in the next session, you begin to plan the next exposure.

> Remember to link behavioral change to cognitive change. "What does your success mean about you?"

RELAXATION TECHNIQUES

Relaxation techniques are a powerful tool for combating anxiety and tension (Benson, 1975; Jacobson, 1974). Remember that thoughts, feelings, and behavior are all related. Therefore, anxious thoughts, feelings, and behavior come together as a package. It is impossible for the body to be both tense and relaxed at the same time, so helping the body to relax is a behavioral way to also change anxious feelings and thoughts.

There are four main relaxation techniques:

- Progressive relaxation
- Breathing exercises
- Meditation
- Imagery

Below is an example of how these techniques could be introduced in session. After the idea of relaxation techniques has been introduced to the student, you will describe the specifics of the techniques that you will be trying with the student. Remember to first teach the technique in a session and have the student practice the new skill with you. After the student has learned the basics of using relaxation in session, the student should practice using the techniques at other times. Overall, the student will first practice the techniques in situations that are not stressful so that the skills are strengthened. Then, over time, the student will start using the techniques to relax in situations that are stressful. If a student immediately starts trying to relax in stressful situations, he is unlikely to have early successes, which could lead the student to give up before he has really built the skills.

CLINICIAN: David, we've been talking about the fact that sometimes you get stressed out or anxious and react in ways that end up not working for you, right?

DAVID: Yeah. That's when I kind of freak out and overreact. The thing is, I can't help it! People criticize me or pick on me, and I just lose it.

CLINICIAN: You've mentioned before that it feels like you can't get any control over those reactions, but I have some techniques that we could practice that might help. Would you be willing to give some of those techniques a try?

DAVID: Sure, I guess. I don't know if it will work, though.

CLINICIAN: Fair enough. I think it's great that you're willing to give it a try even though you're not sure it will work! So, the main thing I want to think about with you is relaxation. Do you have things that you already do to relax?

DAVID: Yeah. I listen to music to relax sometimes.

CLINICIAN: That's a great example! One of the things that can be tricky, though, is when you need to relax but you're in a situation where you can't walk away to listen to music or do some of the other things people might do.

DAVID: Like if I need to relax, but I'm in class or something?

CLINICIAN: Exactly. So I'd like to tell you about a couple of other ways you could relax, and then I'll have you try them out and tell me what you think.

DAVID: OK . . . but I don't really understand how that will help with how I react kind of strongly in those situations.

CLINICIAN: Then I'm glad you told me that! The way our bodies work is that they can't be *tense* and *relaxed* at the same time. Muscles, for example, are either tight or loose, but they can't be both at the same time. By using relaxation skills, we can keep our bodies relaxed and loose. So, if you think about how the cognitive model tells us that thoughts, feelings, and behavior are all related, what do you think happens if we can keep our bodies more relaxed?

DAVID: I guess I feel more relaxed emotionally, too?

CLINICIAN: Exactly! And if you're feeling physically and emotionally more relaxed, what do you think happens when you end up in a situation where you'd normally get stressed out and react in a way that doesn't end up working for you?

DAVID: I guess I end up not reacting as strongly or maybe not as quickly.

CLINICIAN: You've got it. So, does that sound like something worth trying?

DAVID: Sure.

CLINICIAN: Great. There are four different techniques we can talk about, and then you can try them out and see what works best for you. Let's talk about progressive relaxation, breathing exercises, meditation, and imagery.

The clinician can then introduce each of the following techniques and have David try them in the session. They will continue to practice the skills in session until David has learned them well enough to try them at home. You may decide to make a recording of yourself talking through one of the scripts in the Appendices so that students can listen to it at home to practice, or David may prefer to practice without the audio. The Internet offers many different audio clips with relaxation exercises, so you and David may also find clips there that he likes to use to practice. The following are four relaxation techniques most commonly used in the schools.

Progressive relaxation is a systematic way of tensing and relaxing groups of muscles to relax the body (Jacobson, 1974). As with any of the cognitive or behavioral strategies, learning progressive relaxation requires a lot of practice. Students are asked to practice relaxing at a time when they are not tense, like an hour before bedtime each night. This gives the student a chance to learn relaxation without having to fight against anxiety and tension. Once the skill is mastered, the student can use progressive relaxation at stressful times to relax the body, and in turn experience less cognitive and emotional stress. An example of a relaxation script is also included in Appendix 4.6 at the end of the book. You may find that students respond particularly well to a recording of your voice reading the script, because you are a voice they associate with feeling relaxed and safe. A time-saver is to make one recording of yourself reading a script of your choice, and then make copies of the recording for students to play. Below, a clinician introduces progressive relaxation to Anjanae as a technique to help her fall asleep at night when she is worrying.

CLINICIAN: One of the relaxation techniques that might be particularly helpful for you is progressive relaxation, which is a way of relaxing one group of muscles at a time until your body feels really relaxed. People usually use progressive relaxation to either relax before something stressful (like giving a speech) or to fall asleep at night.

ANJANAE: That sounds great! I worry a lot if I have to talk in front of the class, and it always takes me a long time to fall asleep at night.

CLINICIAN: Well, then it sounds like this might be a good thing for us to practice together. I have a script I'm going to read to you, and it will walk you through the different things you're going to do to relax. Let's try it together in here and see how it works for you. Maybe you could also take it home and try it as a practice, too. What do you think?

ANJANAE: It seems like it's worth a try.

CLINICIAN: Great! OK, get nice and comfortable there in your chair, and I'll start reading it to you. Ready?

Breathing exercises help the student to slow down, control his breathing, and get enough oxygen to help his body relax (Benson, 1975). When a student is anxious or tense, he is likely to breathe more shallowly and quickly, which sends signals to the nervous system that there is danger nearby, triggering a type of fight-or-flight response. Slowing the breathing will help to reverse these messages to the nervous system, soothing the fight-or-flight response. A student learns to breathe slowly in through the nose and out through the mouth. A deep breath should cause the student's belly to expand, as the diaphragm pulls air into the student's lungs. If only the upper chest is expanding on the deep breaths, then the student is not completely filling his lungs and getting the full benefit of deep breathing. Once a student is aware of his breath during stressful situations and makes sure the breathing is deep and slow, he can use this method to effectively reduce anxiety and tension. As with progressive relaxation, there are many scripts and audio files of breathing exercises on the Internet to choose from. A script of a breathing exercise is also included in Appendix 4.7 at the end of the book. Below, the clinician introduces breathing exercises to David as a way to relax in stressful situations.

CLINICIAN: OK, David, I'd like to try some breathing exercises. These are one of the ways I mentioned that can help you relax, and that are subtle enough that you can do them in class, in the cafeteria, at the mall, or anywhere else you need to relax. Ready to give it a try?

DAVID: OK.

CLINICIAN: Great. Remember how we were talking about ways to help your body relax so that your thoughts and feelings are more relaxed, too?

DAVID: Yeah, I remember.

CLINICIAN: Good. I'm going to read you a script that will help you to do some breathing exercises.

DAVID: But I breathe all day long. I even breathe when I sleep! So why do I need you to tell me how to breathe?

CLINICIAN: This is actually a different kind of breathing than what you usually do. This way, you're paying more attention to your breathing so that it's nice and slow, with deep breaths. You'll get a lot of oxygen into your body without hyperventilating, so that your body will slow down. Can we give it a try?

DAVID: Yeah, OK.

CLINICIAN: Good. So, get nice and comfortable and I'll read this to you. You can just follow along and see how it works for you. Then, maybe we can set you up to practice it at home, too. Let's give it a try now and see how it goes in here.

Meditation is a way of clearing the mind so that both one's thoughts and one's heart rate slow down (Hayes, Follette, & Linehan, 2004). Meditation can be helpful for students who are having racing thoughts, whether anxiety, depression, stress, or other issues are at the root of the distress. Anjanae was told by her clinician about meditation as another way to focus and relax at night, because now she often lays awake for up to 2 hours worrying about her grades, her family, and safety issues in her neighborhood. She and her clinician spent time in session planning the best way for Anjanae to try meditation at home, thinking about a good time and place to be able to sit quietly for a few minutes. They also practiced meditation in the session, focusing on a peaceful picture that the clinician has on her wall. Anjanae had to work hard to find a quiet place to meditate in her house, but she's found that she can close herself in her mother's bedroom while her mother is at work. Anjanae lights a candle in the room for some calming light and makes herself comfortable in a chair near a painting of a big open field. She concentrates on the scene in the painting, emptying her mind of any other thoughts or worries. If she realizes that her mind has drifted back to worries, she remembers that her clinician taught her to not to be angry at herself. Instead, she just moves her concentration back to the painting. Her thoughts start to slow down, and as they do, Anjanae's body relaxes and she begins to feel more peaceful. On some nights, she concentrates on the candle flame instead of the picture, but the picture is her favorite focus point. Regardless of what she focuses on, the key to meditation is to focus on one point and let any other distractions pass out of your mind. If Anjanae catches herself and realizes that her mind has wandered, she recognizes this and redirects her attention to her focus point, without judging herself or getting frustrated that her mind wandered. It is not unusual for her to have to redirect her thoughts several times, which she reminds herself is just part of the process of meditation. Once she feels relaxed and calm (usually about 10 minutes), she gets up from the chair, blows out the candle, and heads to her bed. Anjanae has been falling asleep much more quickly since she started meditating at night.

Imagery is a relaxation technique that has some similarity to meditation (Hayes et al., 2004). To use imagery, a student begins, as Anjanae did, by finding a private, quiet place and getting comfortable. However, instead of focusing on something like a picture or a candle, for imagery the student will choose a relaxing setting and imagine the sights, sounds, smells, sensations, and tastes that go with that setting. By using all of the senses as part of the imagery, the student's imagination takes over so that she almost feels like she is in the relaxing setting. Often, the most effective settings to imagine are places that students have been, because they will most easily be able to imagine the sights, sounds, smells, sensations, and tastes in that setting. However, students can choose any setting that will help them to relax, as long as they are able to imagine all of the details they need to really immerse themselves in the setting. As with the other relaxation techniques, there are many websites that offer streaming audio that can help the student to picture a relaxing place. Below, a clinician suggests imagery to Alfred as a way to relax and focus when he is feeling frustrated after a wrestling match.

CLINICIAN: It makes a lot of sense to me that you still feel wound up and agitated after wrestling—especially if the match didn't go completely the way you might have wanted. Let's see if we can think of a way to help you relax after the match, OK?

ALFRED: OK. That could really help, because otherwise I end up going home and snapping at my brother for little stuff.

CLINICIAN: OK, then let's try this instead. One good way to unwind is to take a kind of mini-vacation in your mind. As an example, can you name a place where you can imagine yourself being, where you would be really relaxed? It should be somewhere really peaceful and safe, and it can be somewhere you've actually been or somewhere you'd like to go. The most important thing is that it should be somewhere you can imagine in detail. Can you think of a place like that?

Alfred: Yeah. Last summer, I went to the beach with my cousin. Most of the time wasn't relaxing, or at least not the way you're talking about. We had too much fun for that! But there was one morning when I woke up before everybody else, right as the sun was coming up. I couldn't fall back asleep, so I got up and walked over to the beach from our hotel. I sat and watch the sun come up over the water, which was pretty cool.

CLINICIAN: That's a great example! What I want you to do is close your eyes and try to remember that whole scene, almost like you're watching a movie in your mind. If you were going to watch a movie of the peaceful part, where would you start?

ALFRED: I guess I'd start after I got to the beach.

CLINICIAN: OK, then close your eyes and imagine yourself standing on the edge of the beach. I want you to try to use all five of your senses to think about the answers to my next questions, but you don't need to answer them out loud. What do you see? Look all around in your mind at the water, the sky, the sand . . . (*pause for a moment*) What do you hear? (*pause*) Can you feel the breeze on your skin and the sand under your feet? (*pause*) What do you smell? The ocean water, or anything else? (*pause*) And can you taste anything, like the salt in the air? (*pause*) Try to remember what you saw as you stood on the beach, watching the sun slowly rise over the water (*pause*) Remember the colors in the sky, the feel of the wind and the sand, the smell of the ocean (*pause*) Keep imagining each moment of the sunrise, remembering to use all of your senses (*pause*) When you have seen the whole movie of the sunrise, I want you to take three very slow, deep breaths, and then when you're ready, open your eyes . . .

ALFRED: (*After a few minutes, opens his eyes.*)

CLINICIAN: How are you feeling right now?

ALFRED: That was actually pretty cool. I wasn't sure it was going to work, but I do feel different now. I feel more relaxed and kind of quieter.

CLINICIAN: I think that's really great. How about if we think about ways that you could do that kind of imagery in other situations, like on the bus on the way home from wrestling practice?

ALFRED: That sounds good to me.

SUPPORTING EVIDENCE

At the end of Chapter 3, we introduced the research support for the relationship between clients' thoughts and their symptoms, ranging from depression to substance abuse to post-traumatic stress disorder. Behavioral techniques are used to facilitate change in thoughts, much like the cognitive techniques in the previous chapter.

Behavioral experiments function much like some of the cognitive strategies in the previous chapter, in that they are active, behavior-based ways to test out beliefs and assumptions. Behavioral activation has been shown to significantly decrease symptoms of depression (Syzdek, Addis, & Martell 2010) and, in fact, sustained focus on behavior change in time-limited treatments has been shown to be a powerful intervention for depression (Coffman, Martell, Dimidjian, Gallop, & Hollon, 2007). The use of replacement behavior originally hails from applied behavior analysis (ABA) (Baer, Wolf & Risley, 1968, 1987). ABA was very behaviorally focused, identifying undesirable behaviors and the needs that were met through those behaviors and then reinforcing more desirable behaviors. The use of replacement behavior in CT focuses not only on changing the behaviors, but also on the cognitions that explain or maintain the behaviors.

Exposures are a widely used and well supported intervention technique for a number of anxiety disorders (Albano & Kendall, 2002; Ollendick & King, 1998). Table 4.2 provides a few of the many examples of research that has shown the efficacy of exposure for anxiety.

SUMMARY

Behavioral techniques offer a second angle for intervening in the triangle of thoughts, feelings, and behavior. These techniques (behavioral experiments, behavioral activation, safety plans, hope kits, replacement behavior, exposure and relaxation techniques) can be a powerful part of your cognitive work with students. There is not a one-size-fits-all way to plan behavioral interventions because each intervention should be tailored for your student's individual strengths and needs. Once the individual plan has been made, you and the student have the opportunity to learn a great deal, regardless of the specific outcome of the plan.

Remember that behavioral strategies are an important part of CT and not just a supplement to it. Treatment plans are often anchored to behavior patterns that are causing problems for students, and these strategies can help to make major changes in those behaviors. Asking the student to *reflect* on their experiences with behavioral interventions—both successes and problems—and consider how those experiences *relate to their thought patterns and beliefs* is a vital component to using behavioral techniques. Each behavioral strategy should lead to learning about the thought and belief anchors for treatment, helping move students toward seeing themselves as competent, capable, and worthwhile.

TABLE 4.2. Empirical Support for the Use of Exposure

Disorder	Studies supporting exposure use
Panic disorder with or without agoraphobia	Beck, Emery, & Greenberg (1990); Landon & Barlow (2004)
Posttraumatic stress disorder	Foa et al. (1999, 2005); Foa, Rothbaum, Riggs, & Murdock (1991); Resick, Nishith, Weaver, Astin, & Feuer (2002)
Generalized anxiety disorder	Kendall et al. (2005); Ladouceur, Dugas, Freeston, Léger, Gagnon, & Thibodeau (2000)
Obsessive–compulsive disorder	Franklin, Abramowitz, Kozak, Levitt, & Foa, (2000); Van Oppen, de Haan, Van Balkom, & Spinhoven (1995); Foa, Steketee, Grayson, Turner, & Latimer (1984); Foa, Steketee, & Milby (1980); Foa, Steketee, Turner, & Fischer (1980)
Social phobia	Davidson et al. (2004); Kendall et al. (2005); Heimberg et al. (2000); Cottraux et al. (2000)
Specific phobias	Gotestam & Hokstad (2002); Öst, Alm, Brandberg, & Breitholtz (2001); Muhlberger, Wiedemann, & Pauli (2003); Willumsen, Vassend, & Hoffart (2001)

READER ACTIVITY: BEHAVIORAL INTERVENTION

Behavioral interventions may be familiar to some clinicians who are just beginning their CT training, but many clinicians discover that even if they already use some behavioral techniques, CT frames those interventions in a slightly different light. Choose any one of the behavioral interventions described in this chapter. Then design a behavioral intervention that would target issues faced by a student with whom you have worked.

What is the student's thought, belief, or problematic behavior that is being targeted with this intervention?

_____

_____

_____

_____

_____

Which intervention would you choose for this student, and why?

_____

_____

_____

_____

How would you design the intervention? Remember, in a real situation, you would collaboratively design the intervention with very active participation and input from the student. However, for this exercise, imagine the kinds of suggestions the student might make while planning. What would the student want to do or not want to do? How would you handle that in the planning? Be sure to plan for your intervention to go well, but be prepared in case it does not go as planned.

_____

_____

_____

_____

_____

_____

_____

_____

_____

_____

_____

Imagine that the behavioral intervention went as planned. How would you explore the outcome with the student so that the outcome of the intervention is folded into your cognitive work? Does the outcome support the student's thoughts and beliefs or challenge them?

_____

_____

_____

_____

_____

_____

_____

_____

Now imagine the behavioral intervention did not go as planned. How would you explore this outcome with the student so that the outcome of the intervention is folded into your cognitive work? Does the outcome support the student's thoughts and beliefs or challenge them?

_____

_____

_____

_____

_____

_____

_____

_____

On the basis of each of the outcomes above, what would you plan as a next step in helping the student to work on the targeted thoughts, beliefs, or behaviors?

_____

_____

_____

_____

_____

_____

_____

_____

CHAPTER 5

Making Cognitive Therapy Happen in the Schools

OTHER UNIQUE CHALLENGES AND REWARDS OF THE SCHOOL SETTING

CT has been successfully adapted for use in a school setting, but some unique challenges and rewards to using CT with students remain . Counseling services within schools typically have a very large caseload with very limited staff. The staff must find a way to fit mental health services into a busy academic day, which results in sessions that are much shorter than the typical "50 minute hour, once per week" type of therapy. In addition to these ongoing short sessions, many school clinicians find themselves managing a large number of crisis sessions each week. Clinicians also have limited access to students' families and other home-based information. Finally, resources (including space) in school mental health settings are often quite limited. Given these challenges, school-based clinicians may feel challenged to provide effective CT to their students. However, working in a school setting also offers some distinct advantages over other settings.

In a school, clinicians have access to information about an adolescent's academic and social functioning that they might not have in any other situation. School clinicians can observe a student's interactions with peers and staff, and they can get valuable information about grades, homework, classroom behavior, and other important academic issues. In addition, clinicians have regular access to the students who attend school regularly. Therefore, a clinician may see a student two or three times per week, for 30 minutes each. Schools also offer a team environment in which the clinician is working with other professionals, all focused on supporting the same group of adolescents. The opportunity to work with the school staff, with all of the

CT is particularly well suited to the challenges and advantages of a school setting.

diverse skills and backgrounds they bring with them, is a major advantage of the school setting. Ideally, you may use your role as the clinician to educate staff on thinking patterns and other CT concepts during inservices or other appropriate outlets. Of course, the level of support for such training will vary from school to school. From the principal to the lunch support staff to teachers, each staff member you can teach to think in a CT manner can support the changes you are encouraging in your students. Finally, clinicians are able to offer their students a "safe place" in the school, which can be rewarding for both the student and the clinician.

On the other hand, experienced clinicians are not surprised to hear that students sometimes take advantage of the "safe place" in the clinician's office to avoid other school activities. Students may come to the clinician's office to avoid a class they dislike, a presentation they are scheduled to give, or a pop quiz. Often, this behavior is not an "either or" situation—students may genuinely need to visit the clinician's office, but strategically schedule that visit during a class or they wish to avoid. (This behavior may even be a compensatory strategy for some students!) The clinician can leverage this motivation and use it to the advantage of the student and the clinician by requiring some effort on the part of students. For example, Presession Quick Sheets can be mandated for students who arrive for counseling, limited a sensitivity to the needs, abilities, and situation of the student. These types of expectations may reduce the number of students who come to the clinician's office to escape, when they realize that participation in real counseling work is expected of them.

CT can work particularly well within these challenges and advantages. For example, you can make your own observations of the student in academic and social settings to help support the student in testing beliefs. Schools also present the opportunity for the clinician to work together with other school staff-support interventions, so that the student receives support beyond your sessions. CT is present focused, goal oriented, and anchored to specific problematic thought and behavior patterns, which helps students and clinicians to be productive and to focus their time together. Finally, CT has a distinct session structure that can help clinicians and students to accomplish more work in less time than they might in a more unstructured therapy.

GOAL SETTING

Situations or problems that are in the here and now are usually the focus of CT, which makes this type of counseling a particularly good fit for a school setting. Treatment is goal oriented, with the clinician and student working together to define

> **Clear, collaboratively set goals help to keep counseling moving forward, and they can also help you to know when counseling is finished.**

goals, work toward those goals, and determine when the goals have been met. Goals are set early in treatment;the clinician and student can then use those goals as a measuring stick for how much progress is being made in counseling. The goals can also help to define the topics of discussion for a session (which we will discuss next), and they should tie directly in to the case conceptualization that you develop for each student. Sessions are anchored to specific problematic thoughts, behaviors, and beliefs that interfere with the student meeting these goals, and these anchors will appear in most sessions over time. For example, one of the anchors for Alfred's counseling may be his underlying belief that he has to act aggressively whenever someone challenges him so that he does not look weak. When Alfred comes to session and presents a situation in which that belief was triggered, leading him to get into a fight, the clinician will address that pattern. The clinician would simultaneously:

1. Show how that belief, and the resulting compensatory strategy (throwing the first punch in a fight) leads to ongoing problems for Alfred.
2. Help Alfred to solve his current problem (getting detention, which will further interfere with wrestling team participation).
3. Teach Alfred skills to prevent this thought and behavior anchor from getting in the way of reaching his goals.

Below is an example of a clinician setting goals with Anjanae. Notice how collaboratively the clinician works to set the goals, as she encourages Anjanae to actively take the lead in the decisions. Although clinicians may sometimes get input from other staff members, or even parents, about what they think treatment goals should be, it is vital that the student be on board with any goals that are set. If the treatment goals are not ones the student values, she probably will not engage in the treatment very effectively. However, the reality of counseling in a school is that a clinician may be juggling the requirements or expectations of a number of people or groups. A school clinician may be working to simultaneously meet the needs or requirements of

- The student
- Teachers
- Parents and other family members
- The principal
- Special services teams in the school (including an individualized education plan)
- The school district
- Local, state, and federal laws (including the Individuals with Disabilities Act, the 504 plan, and so on)

Juggling these sometimes competing demands is no small matter, and an overall strategy for managing these complexities is far beyond the scope of this book. However, from a CT perspective, it is vital that the student be on board with the stated goals of counseling. If the student does not engage in the setting and strive toward counseling goals, it is very unlikely that meaningful progress will be made on the goals. Therefore, finding a way to frame the treatment goals in the context of the student's current problems will encourage the student to fully participate in counseling.

We find a three-stage process (Figure 5.1) to be very helpful in setting counseling goals. We encourage clinicians to begin with a problem list, move on to explain the cognitive model, and then create a goal list. These steps may take two to three sessions to complete,

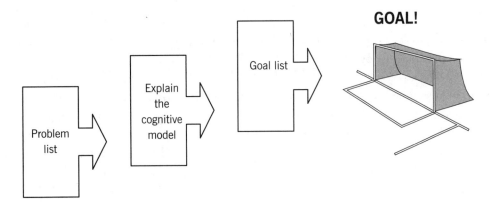

FIGURE 5.1. Three-stage process for setting goals.

but the time is well invested in joining with the student, explaining the model that will form the structure for counseling, and then creating a concrete goal list that the student supports.

Problem List

In a first session, it is clinically important to hear all of the problems that the student is bringing with her. If you begin counseling by listening to all of the student's problems and expressing empathy, you will go a long way toward having the student feel understood and cared for. The list may be longer than can realistically be managed in counseling, but it will give the student time to share all of the problems in a supportive and caring environment.

Review the vignettes from Chapter 1 and choose one student to consider closely. What would be on the problem list he or she would be likely to bring to counseling? How would you listen and communicate empathy to that student during the session?

_____

_____

_____

_____

_____

_____

The Cognitive Model

After the student has had the chance to share an overview of all of the stressors and problems she has, you will transition to talking about the cognitive model. This transition may not happen until your second meeting, but it is important to share the cognitive model early in counseling so that the student understands the framework for the rest of your meetings. Transition naturally from the problem list to the cognitive model, using a narrative similar to the one presented below.

> "Thank you so much for sharing all of that with me. I can really see that you have a lot of concerns that you're dealing with, and it sounds like they are really weighing you down and getting in the way of you living your life the way you want to. I'm really going to want to hear more about those things, but before I do, I want to tell you about something called the cognitive model. The cognitive model is what I use to help me understand students and the issues they are dealing with in their lives. I'd like to tell you how it works, so that, as we're working together, you will be able to understand why I am asking certain questions, or suggesting certain things for you to try. Can we talk about that for a minute?"

How would you introduce the cognitive model to the student whose problem list you created? Would you say something like the script above, or would you have a different way to explain why you wanted to switch from talking about problems to talking about the cognitive model?

_____

_____

_____

_____

_____

_____

This is also a good time to review the cognitive model, including the rollercoaster story and the alternative to the rollercoaster story that you wrote about in Chapter 1. Now that you have learned more about the cognitive model, does the story you wrote still make sense? If not, write a new story below to explain how thoughts, not situations, lead to feelings. Be sure to include the details you have learned about the cognitive model from the rest of your work in this book.

_____

_____

_____

_____

_____

_____

Goal List

Once you understand the problem list and the student understands the cognitive model, you will start to create a goal list. The goal list should be created by the third session, ideally. Although the student may have presented a long list of goals, it may not be possible to address more than one or two major goals at a time in counseling. Therefore, you will help the student to prioritize goals that can realistically be addressed in school counseling, that do not conflict with the requirements or expectations of the many individuals and agencies who may be invested in the counseling goals, and that will help the student to feel like meaningful change has occurred. Goal setting should include very specific and concrete measures of progress. The clinician and student should think about the following types of questions:

- "How will we know if you are meeting your goals?"
- "What would it look like if you met your goals?"
- "How would your life be different? What would you be doing differently?"
- "If someone else were to look at you now, and then look at you after you met your goals, what would he or she see that was different?

Below, Anjanae and her clinician work to set goals for counseling. This conversation takes place in the third session, after the problem list has been shared, the clinician has expressed empathy and warmth toward Anjanae and her problems, and the cognitive model has been described.

CLINICIAN: You've told me a lot about what is going on in your life, and I really appreciate how honest you've been with me. I know it can be hard to talk about that stuff with someone you really don't know very well.

ANJANAE: Yeah. That's all right.

CLINICIAN: Well, it sounds like you have a lot of problems that are really hard for you to deal with. I want to make sure that I have a good sense of what you want to get out of meeting with me, so that I can be as helpful as possible. I'd like to make a list of what you're hoping to accomplish here, just so we have a good sense of where we're headed. We'll also talk about how we will know if we are meeting your goals. Does that sound OK?

ANJANAE: I guess so. I mean, aren't you gonna tell me what I'm supposed to do about all of this? Isn't that your job? If I knew what to do, I wouldn't be here! Weren't you listening to me?

CLINICIAN: I really see my job as being here to help you decide what you want to do. I don't have all the answers. What I can do is to help you decide what the right answers are for you. That would start with me knowing what you really want and need. I have some ideas from what you've told me so far, but I want to make sure I'm on the right track.

ANJANAE: OK. What do you think so far?

CLINICIAN: Well, I know that you want to decide about the next steps about your pregnancy and finding a way to reach your goals for high school and college, about managing your responsibilities at home, and about worrying when you're trying to sleep at night. You also said that you're worried about your grades, and that part of that is because you have a lot of responsibilities at home. Did I get all of the really important concerns?

ANJANAE: Yes. It sounds like a lot when you say it all together like that!

CLINICIAN: Well, there are a lot of things to manage in your life right now. I want to make sure that we do a really good job with the problems that would make the most difference to you, though. What I'd like to do is figure out the one or two most important ones for you and focus on those. Are there one or two problems that, if we really helped you to figure out, you would feel like we had done something worthwhile?

ANJANAE: Yeah. How am I ever gonna be able to have a life, with college and a good career, now that I'm pregnant? I need to figure out how to handle that situation before I deal with anything else.

CLINICIAN: OK. It sounds like that goes on your goal list. Is there anything else we need to make sure we deal with so that you can feel like you're doing OK?

ANJANAE: My grades. Especially now that I'm pregnant, I don't know how I'm ever going to pull my grades up so I can get into a good college.

CLINICIAN: OK. That's two big goals. If we were to help you sort out a plan for dealing with your pregnancy and help you to feel good about how you were doing academically, would that feel like we had really made progress on important goals?

ANJANAE: Yeah.

CLINICIAN: OK. Now let's figure out how we'll both know when you're doing better on those two goals. Which one do you want to start with?

ANJANAE: The pregnancy. Definitely.

CLINICIAN: OK. How will you know that you're making progress in dealing with the fact that you're pregnant? What would I be able to see that was different? Or what would you be doing that was different?

ANJANAE: For starters, I would have already made a decision about what to do. I mean, it's really gonna mess up my plans if I try to raise this baby, but I can't imagine giving it up for adoption, and my faith rules out any other options.

CLINICIAN: Yes, I can definitely see that figuring out what to do is going to be really hard, but I promise that I'll be right here to help you with that. If you make a decision about what to do, will that be enough for you to feel like the situation is under control?

ANJANAE: No! Even after I figure out what to do, I will still have to figure out *how* to do it. I mean, I want to go to college! Can I do that as a single mom? But what other choice do I have?

CLINICIAN: It sounds like what you're saying is that you want to make a decision and then have a plan in place for how to make your decision work. Is that right?

ANJANAE: Yes. That sounds pretty good.

CLINICIAN: OK. I'll write that down. And then for the other issue you mentioned, your grades, how will we know if you've reached your *goal* there so it doesn't repeat?

ANJANAE: I will have straight A's.

CLINICIAN: Wow, that's a really high goal! What if for now, I write down that you will be getting grades that you feel good about. Maybe we can spend some more time talking about what kind of grades you could feel good about. Would that be OK?

ANJANAE: Yeah, I guess so.

CLINICIAN: Thanks. I really appreciate your being flexible about that. I hope that the reason I wanted to tweak the wording like that will make a little more sense as we go along. So, if we are working toward those two goals, will you feel like we're being productive in counseling and helping you with the most important concerns for now?

ANJANAE: Yes. That sounds pretty good.

With this goal list in mind, Anjanae and her clinician can focus on helping her to meet her goals. As time passes and situations in Anjanae's life change, the goal list may change, too. Anjanae may also come to some sessions wanting to talk about goals that are not on her original goal, which will be perfectly fine. The goal list is meant to give direction to the counseling work, but not to be rigid or restrictive. Remember that, along with the list, the clinician will keep in mind the anchor behaviors and thoughts—the patterns that have been getting in the way of Anjanae meeting her goals. For example, Anjanae revealed a little bit about one of her beliefs while she was goal setting. Did you catch it? If so, write it below.

_____

_____

_____

If you caught Anjanae's thought about straight A's being the only way to have "good grades," then you're really on top of things! Over time, the clinician could anchor counseling to her pattern of having thinking traps like "Shoulds" and "A Perfect Disaster"—her belief that anything less than straight A's is a failure. As a student with a 3.7 GPA, particularly with all the stress she has been experiencing, Anjanae has admirable grades!

SESSION STRUCTURE

In Chapter 1, we briefly introduced one of the unique features of CT: the structured way in which each session unfolds. The session structure creates a sense of hope for students, communicating that the problems they face can be tackled in a systematic way, rather than overwhelming them. In addition, structure can help to keep therapy organized, on track, and efficient, which is particularly important in the shorter sessions that are typical in a school setting. In our experience, students come to expect the structure as part of the routine. In training school clinicians, we noticed that some clinicians have automatic thoughts about using a structure in counseling. Were you able to catch any of your own automatic thoughts? If so, please write them below.

_____

_____

_____

_____

_____

Some therapists catch thoughts like, "Being so structured in session may alienate the students" or "This sounds too rigid." If this is the case for you, we invite you to try the CT structure for 6 months as a behavioral experiment. Six months from now, come back to the automatic thoughts you wrote down and check whether your initial thoughts were accurate. In looking at your thoughts, we hope you will revisit this text and ask yourself:

- "Did I use the techniques as they were described?"
- "Were the outcomes what I expected?"
- "What, if anything, was different from what I expected?"

The structure, which may feel strange at first, is useful for many reasons. It helps optimize your time with the student by defining and focusing on issues; it demonstrates a pragmatic way to understand, address, and solve problems; and it assures that counseling sessions are being used by students who want to work with you to address problems. (Often, those students who merely want to miss algebra will be reluctant to invest the energy in following this structure). There are five structured tasks in a CT session: review of the Presession Quick Sheet, agenda setting, discussion of agenda items, summary/feedback, and homework planning (see Figure 5.2).

Some clinicians are initially put off by this list, thinking, "How can I possibly do all of that in one 30-minute session?" In our experience, having this kind of structure helps clinicians and students to make the most of that 30-minute session. Although these times are flexible estimates, the timing of these tasks usually breaks down as follows.

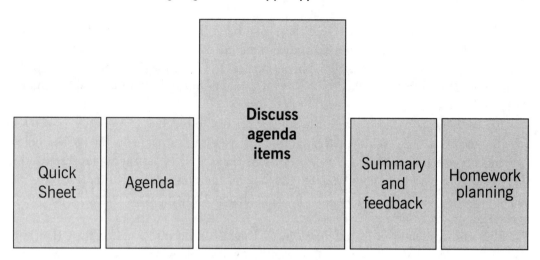

FIGURE 5.2. Five tasks of a CT session.

- Presession Quick Sheet—completed by student before session
- Check-in ⎫
- Agenda ⎭   about 5 minutes
- Discussion of agenda items—   about 20 minutes
- Summary and feedback ⎫
- Homework assignment ⎭   about 5 minutes

Presession Quick Sheet

The Presession Quick Sheet first introduced in Chapter 2, helps students to organize their thoughts about their current mood and situation and their practice in applying CT concepts to their problems. School clinicians we have trained have told us that keeping a stack of Quick Sheets in the area where students wait for their meetings makes their use simple and convenient. Students take a moment prior to the meeting to use the Quick Sheet to organize their thoughts, which facilitates a quick start to the session.

Check-In and Presession Quick Sheet Review

In the beginning of the session, a quick mood check establishes how the student is feeling. An easy way to do this mood check is to review the student's rating on the Quick Sheet. However, if you have chosen not to use the Quick Sheet, simply ask the student to rate, on a 0–10 scale, how he or she is feeling. Regardless of how the rating is obtained, this number can be helpful as a quick reference for the student's state of mind coming into the session, and it can also be tracked over time to show progress and improvement.

A second part of the check-in is to review the student's reactions to the last session. Students may want to talk about something that bothered them about the last session, an idea that was helpful, or an issue that they have been thinking more about between sessions. This feedback can help direct you and your students to issues that are still unresolved or to identify conversations that have been particularly helpful. If a topic comes up that needs more than a few moments of discussion, it should be added to the agenda, which is described below.

Finally, you should check with the student about the practice task that he or she was asked to try between sessions—Although this will be discussed more in the section below, students are asked to do things between sessions that follow up on the topics discussed in the session. The student should check off a box on the Quick Sheet to indicate whether the homework was completed, so a quick check-in about whether it needs to be put on the agenda should be sufficient.

If anything comes up in the check-in that needs to be discussed further, that topic should be added to the agenda. In that way, the session does not get derailed by talking about the items in the check-in, without ever getting to the planned session topics.

Agenda

The agenda is a collaboratively developed road map for the session based on the topics that the student and clinician each want to discuss. In reality, students and clinicians almost always enter a session with "unspoken agenda items" in mind. Alfred may come to the session planning to talk about a fight he had just before school started that morning. As his clinician, you may start the session with an intention to talk with Alfred about his treatment anchor related to acting aggressively so that he will not appear to be weak. Without actually creating an agenda, either or both of these topics may be missed because the conversation never shifted in the right direction. You may spend the whole meeting trying talk with Alfred about his thinking patterns, never knowing that Alfred is feeling frustrated because counseling is not focusing on what he wants to work on. Alternatively, you may feel frustrated because the whole session is spent on Alfred's fight before school, leaving you feeling like sessions are always about dealing with a different daily problem but never making real progress on Alfred's goals. Of course, almost every clinician has had the experience of having a student wait to mention a very important topic until 3 minutes before the session is supposed to end, leaving no time for meaningful discussion. Although having an agenda will not completely prevent that problem, it does create an opportunity for you and the student to prioritize and plan enough session time for the important topics of discussion.

> **The agenda helps clinicians and students to make excellent use of their time in session, creating space for the topics each person wants to address.**

The following conversation is an example of how a clinician could quickly develop an agenda with Alfred. Students come to expect the agenda to be set at the beginning of the session, and they will often come to the session with agenda items in mind. Agenda setting can then happen in less than a minute, as shown in the dialogue that follows. In this way, the student is in control of how much time gets devoted to each topic, but nothing gets accidentally pushed back so that there's a rush at the end to superficially talk about topics and so that none of the topics are unintentionally skipped. The agenda acts as a way to be respectful of the things each of you wanted to talk about in the session, rather than a rigid plan that restricts any topics.

CLINICIAN: So, what would you like to make sure we talk about today?

ALFRED: Well, that guy Mike is looking for a fight, and I think I'm gonna give it to him. I guess we can talk about that.

CLINICIAN: Great. I saw you wrote his name on the Presession Quick Sheet, so I wondered what that was about. I also want to check in about the practice we planned last time we met. I saw that you checked off that you did it—how did it go?

ALFRED: It didn't go that well.

CLINICIAN: OK. Should we put that on our plan for today too?

ALFRED: Sure.

CLINICIAN: Sounds good. Let's also spend a minute talking about progress on the plan for getting you back onto the team, OK? Where should we start?

ALFRED: Let me tell you about this thing with Mike . . .

CLINICIAN: OK. Then do you want to review to the practice or save that for the end?

ALFRED: Let's do that last.

Alfred and his clinician now have a plan for the session (see Figure 5.3), and Alfred was able to choose where to start. If anything comes up during the session that is important to talk about, the clinician should ask Alfred whether he wants to add it to the agenda or make a note of it for the next session. However, if the conversation starts to drift to things that are not important to talk about, like the off-topic chatting that can tempt us and pull us off track during a session, the agenda gives you and the student something to guide you back on track.

The clinician would then keep an eye on the clock to make sure that there was enough time to talk about the topics Alfred prioritized. This conversation might have taken about a minute of the session, and in that time, several things were accomplished. Alfred was able to take charge of the direction of the session and know that the thing he was thinking about (his problem with Mike, his homework not going well) would be discussed. The clinician was able to identify the topics that Alfred wanted to talk about so that he could budget

Agenda		
Fight with Mike	(First)	✓
Take-home practice	(Third)	
Getting back on the team	(Second)	

FIGURE 5.3. Agenda for the session with Alfred.

enough time for them, along with her own agenda item. Without this conversation, they might have spent the whole time talking about Alfred's homework issue and his problem with Mike, and never have gotten to work on getting Alfred back on the wrestling team. Without any agenda at all, the session might have ended up focusing on other topics and totally missed the most important issues of the day.

While you think about the agenda items and listen to the student, try to anchor the discussion to the thinking and behavior patterns that you identified as important in your cognitive conceptualization. This anchoring helps both you and the student know what underlying psychological factors are leading them to think, feel, and behave as they do. Many clinicians find it helpful to use a dry erase board or a paper that shows the student's thinking pattern in relation to their current problem (see Figure 5.4). Doing so helps you make sure you understand the student, which will help assure that your interventions are accurately informed. More important, it gives students a visual description of what is going on when they feel negative emotions. This understanding helps students act as their own clinicians when future problems occur, because they will understand how their thinking patterns and underlying beliefs play a role in the way they think, feel, and behave.

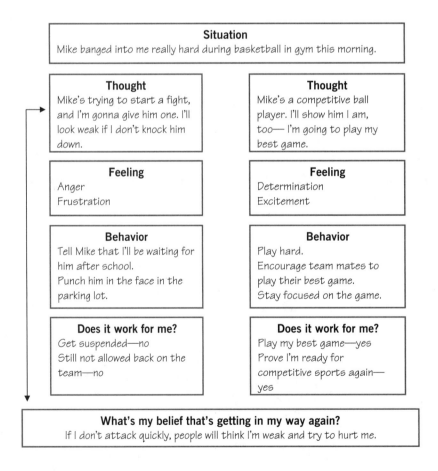

FIGURE 5.4. Illustration of Alfred's thinking patterns about current problems.

Students in Distress

What about when a student arrives in the clinic in emotional distress? Note that this distress would *differ* from a true clinical crisis. Whereas a clinical crisis is a situation such as serious thoughts of suicide or having just been assaulted, a student in emotional distress has a situation that is very distressing to the student but presents no real danger or need for an immediate crisis reaction. For example, a student may be in emotional distress after breaking up with a boyfriend or girlfriend, getting in a pushing match with another student, or failing a test. Some clinicians struggle with these kinds of situations, because when students arrive in distress, the problem can hijack the whole session. Checking in on the agenda, talking about homework, and the other key parts of the session are skipped so that the student and clinician can

> **Sticking to the session structure and framing a "crisis" in terms of the case conceptualization help keep sessions from getting derailed.**

work to put out the fire. When this behavior becomes a pattern, it can become almost impossible to make significant progress in therapy, because sessions are focused on the day's crisis instead of the treatment goals. However, it is quite common for students to arrive at therapy, focused on their distress about a current situation without regard for the bigger picture. Developmentally, adolescents are often uninterested in self-growth, are focused on the present, and want to talk only about their latest problem. Having students look at how their current problem relates to their patterns of thoughts and beliefs creates an opportunity to work on both the immediate situation and the bigger picture issues that create patterns in their lives at the same time. Acknowledging and changing these patterns can help students in the present and in the future.

Although these emotionally distressing situations are very upsetting for the student, they do not require a level of crisis reaction that requires the clinician to reorganize the whole session. (In a true clinical crisis, such as suicidality, having been assaulted, or the like, which are beyond the scope of this text, the clinician should follow the procedures in the clinic for dealing with a crisis.) The Presession Quick Sheet is a particularly helpful tool in these situations. The Quick Sheet leads the student through describing the problem situation, the intensity of her feelings, her thoughts in the situation, and her current plan for dealing with the situation. The form should only take about 2 minutes to complete, and in exchange it provides the student with a moment to calm down and the clinician with a fast way to access the key information about her distress. You may choose to have students complete these Quick Sheets only when they come to a session in distress, or you may have them complete one every time they come to session, on the basis of what you find to be most helpful.

You can review the Quick Sheet as the session begins to get an overview of the student's concerns. Consider how the distressing situation is related to the

- Cognitive conceptualization
- Patterns of thinking
- Student's underlying beliefs
- Treatment goals

} Treatment anchors

Discussing the distressing situation in this way keeps the situation in the larger context and helps you to deal with it without getting sidetracked from the student's ongoing goals. In this way, the situation at hand can be dealt with in session, and the topic is tied to the larger picture of the case conceptualization and treatment goals.

Homework Practices

Students may not be in counseling for more than 30 minutes each week, which makes it very hard to have enough time to make real change if their new skills are not practiced and reflected upon between sessions. In CT, homework is used between sessions to give students an opportunity to refine the strategies discussed in session and test them out in the real world. These out-of-session practices serve several purposes. First, they increase the time that the student is thinking about his work in counseling. Rather than only focusing on change for 30-minute sessions at a time, the student is thinking about change between sessions as he plans and carries out practices. Second, adolescents may initially dismiss skills or strategies developed in sessions. Some adolescents may agree on the surface but really think, "That would never work," or "I would never really do that," while other adolescents may openly state their concerns about applying the skills in the real world. Homework creates an opportunity for testing out the skills to see if they will actually be helpful for the adolescent. Skills that are truly useful can then be applied to the student's life, and skills that are not helpful can be brought back to session for more discussion or changes.

Although some clinicians may hesitate to give therapy homework, counseling in a school setting can lend itself well to incorporating homework. Research suggests that homework in CT may be similar to academic homework given in school in that the ongoing completion of homework can significantly increase how quickly and how well students learn new material and integrate it into their lives (Edelman & Chambless, 1995; Leung & Heimberg, 1996; Neimeyer & Feixas, 1990).

You and the student can work together at the end of each session to plan homework. Homework should always be directly related to the treatment anchors and goals and to the topics covered in the session. A good way to propose the homework is to say something like, "Based on what we've been working on, what would you like to try out this week?" Work with your student to find a task that would be useful and manageable. Setting a date and time that the student will do the assignment can be very helpful, particularly in early sessions, because it will increase the likelihood that the student will actually try the task. In addition, having the student write down the assignment can help her to remember what needs to be done, and to take the task seriously. Whenever possible, it can also be helpful to actually start the homework in the session by beginning the planning, thinking through any barriers, or starting the actual task.

Small or simple completed homework will be more effective than large or complex homework that is never completed.

Homework does not need to be a large task to be effective. Having a smaller, more doable task is much better than a large, complicated task that the student is unlikely to complete. Be sure to set up the task so that you and the student learn something regardless of what happens. If the student did not do the task, what were the obstacles? If she tried the task but it did not work, what happened? If she did a similar task, why did she change, and what did she learn? If she did the task successfully, how can it be extended next week?

Once the task is planned out, it can be helpful to ask students to rate how likely they are to do the assignment, on a scale of 1–100. If students are less than 90% confident that they will do the assignment:

- Work **collaboratively** to choose a practice task.
- Ask them to recall the **reason** that this task was chosen.
- Anticipate any **roadblocks** and problem solve for them.
- **Modify** the task as needed to raise confidence to at least 90%.

At the beginning of the next session, remember to ask about the homework assignment during the check-in or pay attention to the homework check line ("I did _____ did not _____ do my practice task") on the Quick Sheet. Did the student complete the task? Did it go as expected, or were there surprises? What did he or she learn from the experience? We are not suggesting that all of these questions need to be asked, but they provide a framework for what you, as the clinician, want to know about the homework. Generally, homework check-in is very brief. However, if the homework turns out to be an important topic of conversation, it should be added as an agenda topic. Homework tasks are often placed on the agenda for discussion after the check-in is completed. Following up on practices in this way sends the student the message that the practices are important, reinforces the student for practicing, and provides a basis for a discussion of the ongoing issues addressed by the homework.

Note that in this section, homework has also been referred to as a practice, a task, and an assignment. It can also be called a mind-strengthening game, a skill builder, an action plan, or anything else that fits with your style and that of your students. The label placed on these tasks is chosen to facilitate compliance, and you can choose to call them anything that is comfortable for you and the student. Some students do well with calling it "homework," because homework is part of the expectations in school settings. Other students may react poorly to the idea of even more homework, and may react better to the idea of a "practice." Other clinicians just refer to a plan, as in, "So, what's the plan for this week? What would you like to do?" As long as the task and its importance are being communicated, use any label you would like for this (and any other) component of CT.

Feedback and Summary

The last important pieces in structuring a CT session are asking students to provide feedback during the session and summarizing what they got out of the session at the end. A great time to ask for feedback is at the end of one topic and before the transition to the next; another is to check for understanding periodically during the session. Before moving to the new topic, ask students for some feedback about what you've just finished—how did the session feel? Can they summarize the main points? For example:

"So, we've talked about a few different ideas for sorting out the issue you had with Mike. Tell me, what's the final plan? And does that feel like it might work for you? Do you have any hesitations or worries about doing what you've decided?"

Along similar lines, a nice way to tie together feedback, summaries, and homework at the end of the session is to ask the following types of questions at the end of the session:

- "Was this helpful for you today? What was the most helpful part?"
- "Were there any parts that weren't helpful?"
- "Is there anything you wanted to talk about that we didn't get to today? Should we put it on the agenda for next time?"

Followed by:

- "Out of all the ideas we worked on today, what would be the most helpful one for you to practice before I see you again next week?"

Asking students about what they found most helpful, least helpful, or most interesting will help you to modify the focus of treatment and your approach as well as to identify any agenda items that should be changed. Summaries also provide an opportunity for students to reflect on what they have learned or gained in the session. In addition, students will sometimes summarize a session in a way that is completely different from the way that the clinician would summarize it. It can be very informative for clinicians to hear how students perceived the session. If there were misunderstandings or other differences that should be addressed, having students summarize the session will bring those to light and create a chance for them to be discussed. Finally, the homework flows naturally from the summary and feedback and creates an opportunity for students to choose a way to build on the skills they've acquired.

Clinicians sometimes find it easier to think of these components as bookends (see Figure 5.5). Reviewing the Quick Sheet and creating an agenda make up one bookend; asking students to collaboratively create the homework/action plan and provide feedback make up the other bookend. These bookends hold the session together, targeting the problem and showing how it relates to the treatment anchors that are interfering with students reaching their goals.

FAMILIES AND SCHOOL-BASED COGNITIVE THERAPY

Traditionally, outpatient CT therapists working with children and adolescents also work to involve the parents in therapy. Parental beliefs often play a large role in the way a family system functions, and making a change in the whole family can be more effective than making a change in only one member of the family. Belief and behavior patterns can be passed on across generations, as children learn their core beliefs and rules about the world from

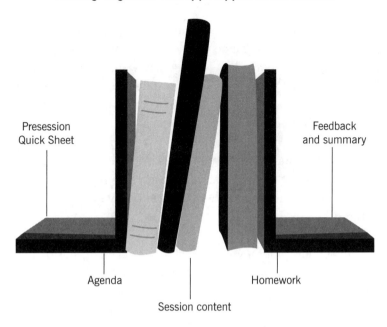

Presession
Quick Sheet

Feedback
and summary

Agenda

Homework

Session content

FIGURE 5.5. Bookends of therapy.

the family that raises them. Parents' beliefs are often communicated to their children both directly and indirectly. For example, a mother may *directly* say to her daughter, "Never trust a man! He will only leave you if you do." Alternatively, a father with a core belief of, "If someone gets angry at me, then it means that the person really doesn't love me," may withdraw whenever his daughter gets angry at him. Even if he never directly voices this belief, his daughter will observe her father's withdrawal and *indirectly* develop her own beliefs from there. For example, she may come to believe that, "I should never show my anger, because it makes people pull away from me. It must make me a bad person to show anger."

When parents are not involved in counseling with their adolescents, the student faces the additional challenge of learning to manage the role of the family's beliefs in his or her own belief system. Therefore, an *ideal* situation would include parents in treatment. However, parental involvement is often *not* possible in school settings. Families, particularly those in low-income urban areas, are often under very high levels

> **Family involvement may not always be possible, but when families are involved, their support can be powerful.**

of stress and may be unable to come to the school to participate. Because of their own past experiences, parents may be uncomfortable in the school setting. They often become used to receiving only "problem" phone calls from the school and may therefore be hesitant to communicate with staff. Work obligations and caring for younger siblings during the day can introduce even more barriers to families coming to the school to participate. Parents may also be hesitant to become involved in their adolescent's treatment because of concerns about a stigma attached to receiving mental health services.

Adolescents may also be hesitant to have their parents involved. As children move into adolescence, they become less focused on family and more focused on their peers, so they may be less interested in having family involvement. Privacy issues can also prevent adolescents from wanting parental involvement. Adolescents may be seeking services for concerns related to their family or home life, or they may want to keep their concerns private from their family. Because laws vary from state to state, be aware of the legal implications in involving a family in an adolescent's treatment in your state. Some states have laws that grant adolescents the right to consent to their own mental health care, which means that those adolescents have a legal right to confidentiality regarding their treatment. Therefore, before trying to involve the family, check your local laws to determine whether you need the adolescent's consent to contact the family. Even if consent is not legally required, obtaining the student's permission to contact his or her family is a very important step to protect your therapeutic relationship.

There are a number of steps you can take to improve the chances that a family may get involved in their adolescent's therapy. First, initiating personal, positive contact with the family through phone calls, e-mail, and letters home can help to overcome parents' expectations that contact from the school indicates bad news. Second, parents can be encouraged to become involved in the homework tasks that an adolescent is carrying out between sessions. These tasks may take place in the home or the neighborhood, and support from parents can be very helpful. Families can also be invited to join a session at school when possible and appropriate. For example, a 30-minute session scheduled during a parent's lunch hour may be an option for some parents, whether in person or on a speakerphone. Also, be sure to have a broad concept of "family" for involvement. Any person who is important to the adolescent and has regular contact with him or her may be appropriate to include. Adolescents may have grandparents, aunts and uncles, cousins, or close family friends who can be supportive of the therapy process. Regardless of who you and the student decide to invite, be sure that you have the proper consent or permission from your student. In the end, your contact with family members may be sporadic or it may be based only on the telephone and e-mails. However, for any students whose families you are able to involve, the potential payoff will truly make it worth your considerable effort.

FUTURE DIRECTIONS: DISSEMINATION

This handbook is one small step in a growing wave of work known as **dissemination**. Dissemination is the process of taking interventions and treatments that were developed in the "ivory tower" of research labs, universities, and other academic settings, and spreading their use into the "real world" of clinical work with students, families, and other clients. Dissemination work is an attempt to bridge the gap between treatments that we know work in controlled settings (based on research studies) and the needs of clinicians in uncontrolled settings, who work with regular people with complex needs. As the bridge between academia and clinical practice is built, researchers and clinicians will continue to collaborate to learn about how these empirically-supported treatments translate into applied settings like the schools. As a clinician who has taken the time to learn more about how CT can be effectively used in a school setting, you are also a part of that growing wave of dissemination and are to be commended for exploring the use of evidence-based interventions in the schools. We hope that this experience has been a positive one, and that you will continue to be at the front of the wave of dissemination work as it builds.

SUPPORTING EVIDENCE

If the idea of dissemination is interesting to you and you would like to learn more about it, many articles are available to help expand your knowledge, among them the following:

- Stirman, S. W., Bhar, S. S., Spokas, M., Brown, G. K., Creed, T. A., Perivoliotis, D., et al. (2010). Training and consultation in evidence-based psychosocial treatments in public mental health settings: The ACCESS model. *Professional Psychology: Research and Practice, 41,* 48–56.
- Beidas, R. S., & Kendall, P. C. (2010). Training therapists in evidence-based practice: A critical review of studies from a systems-contextual perspective. *Clinical Psychology: Science and Practice, 17,* 1–30.

Each of these articles was written with researchers in mind as the intended audience, so you may notice that the language and presentation of the information are quite different from those found in this book. In fact, that difference underscores one part of the disconnect that has existed between research and clinical practice. However, we congratulate you on your interest in bridging that gap, and we encourage you to continue to find ways to integrate empirically supported treatments into your clinical work. In fact, there is evidence that even among clinicians who are all trained in empirically supported therapies, clinicians' personal beliefs about the intervention largely influence which interventions they choose to implement (Forman, Fagley, Steiner & Schneider, 2009).

Some research to study the integration of CT or CBT into school settings has already been done, with promising results. For example, Bernstein and colleagues (Bernstein, Layne, Egan, & Tennison, 2005) found that CBT presented in school-based groups was effective for reducing anxiety in students, particularly when parent groups were also included. CBT has also been successfully implemented in schools to reduce depression (Ruffolo & Fischer, 2009; Shirk, Kaplinski & Gudmundsen, 2009), anger (Smith, Larson, & Nuckles, 2006), attention-deficit/hyperactivity disorder (Bloomquist, August & Ostrander 1991), and a wide variety of other disorders (Gimpel Peacock & Collett, 2010). The skills you have learned in this book will apply to the manuals used in these research studies, as well as your own individually tailored work with your students.

SUMMARY

The structure of a CT session may look challenging when you first consider using it, but that structure can ultimately make your sessions more productive. The goal setting, check-in, agenda, discussion of agenda items, homework assignment, and summary/feedback can help to create a road map for sessions so that threads can be followed from week to week, and students can work on tasks related to those threads between sessions. Treatment anchors are identified, so that when the related thought and behavior patterns arise in session, clinicians help students realize how those patterns can impact the goals they are trying to reach. This format will help students to catch, check, and change the thoughts, behaviors, and underlying beliefs that reoccur and get in their way. Even when a student comes to session with lots of emotion about a situation, the CT structure can help you to incorporate that situation into the bigger picture of therapy. This structure, in combination with the cognitive and behavioral techniques presented in this guide, can be particularly effective in working with the rewards and challenges of a school setting.

Appendices

The Cognitive Model

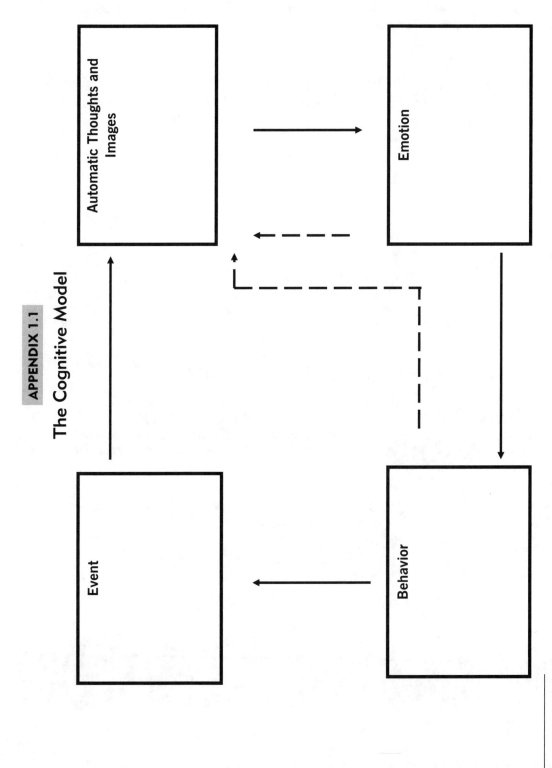

Thinking Traps

The repeat		Thinking that if something happened once, it will always happen the same way.
"It's all about me"		Blaming yourself for bad things that happen, even when they actually have nothing to do with you.
The pessimist		Expecting that things will always turn out for the worst.
Selective sight		Not seeing the good parts of a situation, but picking out all of the dangerous or bad things that could/did happen.
Ignoring evidence		Picking out the evidence that tells you that the worst thing is going to happen, instead of looking at all the evidence to decide what will happen.
The jumper		Jumping to conclusions before getting all the facts about a situation.
The mind reader		Reading minds, but not in a good way—such as deciding that someone is thinking something bad about you without any evidence.
*Should*s		"Should" thinking—"I *should* start a fight with every person who crosses me" or "I *shouldn't* ever get mad."
The crystal ball		Predicting what will happen in the future, and that things will probably go wrong.
A perfect disaster		Thinking that if something is less than perfect, it is a complete failure.

Case Conceptualization

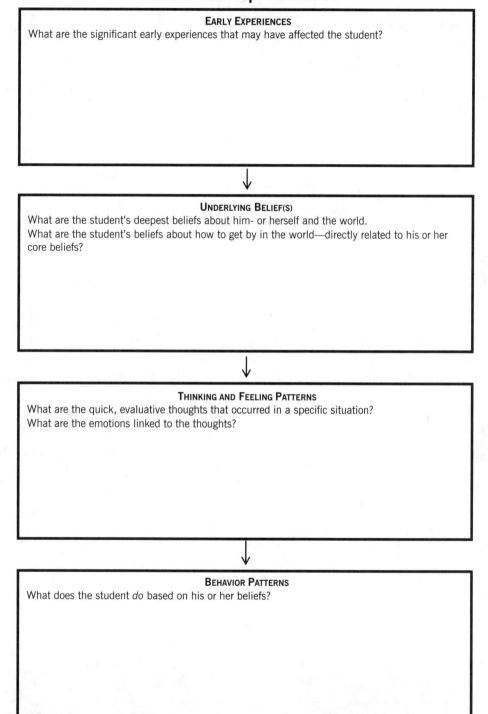

EARLY EXPERIENCES
What are the significant early experiences that may have affected the student?

↓

UNDERLYING BELIEF(S)
What are the student's deepest beliefs about him- or herself and the world.
What are the student's beliefs about how to get by in the world—directly related to his or her core beliefs?

↓

THINKING AND FEELING PATTERNS
What are the quick, evaluative thoughts that occurred in a specific situation?
What are the emotions linked to the thoughts?

↓

BEHAVIOR PATTERNS
What does the student *do* based on his or her beliefs?

Presession Quick Sheet

Today I want to alk about:	I am feeling:	Intensity of feeling:
	Happy	Highest
	Angry	10
	Sad	9
		8
	Worried	7
	Excited	6
What I'm thinking about it is:	Embarrassed	5
		4
	Guilty	3
	Relaxed	2
	Other	1
	_____	Lowest

My best way to deal with it is:

Things I'm thinking about from our last meeting are:

I did ____ did not ____ do my practice task.

Two-Frame Thought Bubble Exercise

In the first box, draw a situation that includes a character with a thought bubble over his or her head. What is that person saying to him- or herself? Be sure to think about how that thought would lead to that person's feelings or behavior in the situation. In the second box, give that character a different thought in the thought bubble. How did the new thought lead to different feelings or behavior?

Thought 1

Thought 2

149

Three-Frame Thought Bubble Exercise

Below, draw a three-box cartoon that shows how a situation, thought, and reaction are related. In Box 1, draw the situation. What is happening? Who is there? What are they doing? In Box 2, draw a picture that includes a thought bubble. What is the main character's automatic thought in the situation? In Box 3, show the main character's reaction. What is the person feeling? How does the person act?

| Situation | Thought | Reaction |

Simple Thought Record

SITUATION

What happened around you just before you felt the way you did?

AUTOMATIC THOUGHT(S)

What thought(s) went through your head?

EMOTION(S)

What emotion(s) did you feel—in one word descriptions?

Thought Record Table

Situation *What happened?*	Thoughts *What was I thinking?*	Feelings *What did I feel?*	Behaviors *What did I do?*

Three C's Thought Record

Time and Day	
Surroundings What was going on around you right before you had a strong feeling?	
Catch Thought What THOUGHT went through your head (remember—usually many words)?	
Feelings What feeling went through your body (remember—usually one word)?	
Check Thought Is the THOUGHT true and/or helpful? True? Helpful?	
Change Thought What THOUGHT would be more true and/or helpful?	

Evaluating Thoughts

Time to check a thought?

✓ What tells you that this thought is true?

✓ What tells you the thought might not be true?

✓ What is the evidence that the thought is true? Not true?

✓ Is there another explanation for what happened?

✓ What is the impact of believing this thought? (pros/cons)

✓ What should you do about it?

✓ If it happened to a friend, what would you say to him or her?

✓ What would your friends say about your thoughts?

✓ Is this thought helpful?

Road Map to Success

Coping Skills

Pleasant Activities List

- Rearrange a room
- Turn up the music and dance
- Volunteer for groups you respect
- Go to a park
- Buy a used musical instrument and learn to play
- Go to a play or concert
- Plan trips or vacations
- Do art or crafts
- Read sacred works (Bible, Torah, Koran...)
- Kiss
- Wear clothes you like
- Read a book or magazine
- Listen to a relaxation CD
- Light candles
- Wear perfume or cologne
- Sit in the sun
- Play a board game
- Finish a difficult task
- Make a list of things you are grateful for
- Take a long bath or shower
- Write a story, poem, music . . .
- Flirt
- Sing or play an instrument
- Go to a religious function
- Learn to say 30 words in another language
- Bake a cake
- Spend time outside
- Wash and style your hair
- Chat with a stranger
- Go to a fair or zoo
- Play with pets
- Listen to music
- Give someone a gift
- Take pictures
- Talk about sports
- Watch or play sports
- Help or protect someone
- Hear jokes (i.e. comedy club, funny movies)
- Spend time somewhere beautiful
- Eat good food
- Sleep late or nap
- Go to a museum or exhibit
- Have a picnic
- Paint a picture
- Be with friends or relatives
- Play a card game
- Talk on the phone
- Daydream
- Go to a movie
- Visit a neighbor
- Play a video game
- Go on the swings in a park
- Reminisce, talk about old times
- Go to a party or give a party
- Volunteer at an animal shelter
- Write in a diary or journal
- Say a prayer
- Meditate
- Get a massage or a back rub
- Go for a walk, hike, or run
- Walk around barefoot
- Pop bubbles in bubble gum
- 10 minutes of deep breathing
- Use your strength
- Go to a barber or beautician
- Be with someone you love
- Rent a movie
- Start a new project
- Go to the library
- Plant seeds in a pot
- Watch people
- Sit in front of a lit fireplace
- Volunteer at a homeless shelter
- Buy flowers for yourself or someone else
- Visit someone who is ill
- Write a letter
- Work out
- Plant or tend a garden
- Hug someone
- Spend time with children
- Stay up late
- Go to a garage sale
- Meet someone new
- Go swimming
- Read cartoons or comic books
- Ride a bike

Reasons for Living

What are the reasons that make you choose to be alive? These reasons for living are different for different people, so it's important to know what they are for you. These reasons may change from time to time, so think about the ones that are your reasons, right now, for being alive.

_____

_____

_____

_____

_____

_____

_____

_____

_____

_____

_____

_____

_____

_____

_____

_____

_____

_____

_____

Pros and Cons List

What are
the good things
about it?

What are the things
that are not good
about it?

Pros	Cons

Fear Hierarchy

Have you ever seen a picture of the pyramids in Egypt? This fear hierarchy is a little bit like those pyramids. You will work with your therapist to make a list of the situations you are worried or nervous about, and then rank them from the easiest to hardest to cope with. Then, you will use your coping skills to conquer the first small step. You can do it! You'll build on your successes and amaze yourself with what you can cope with. Ready? Let's get started!

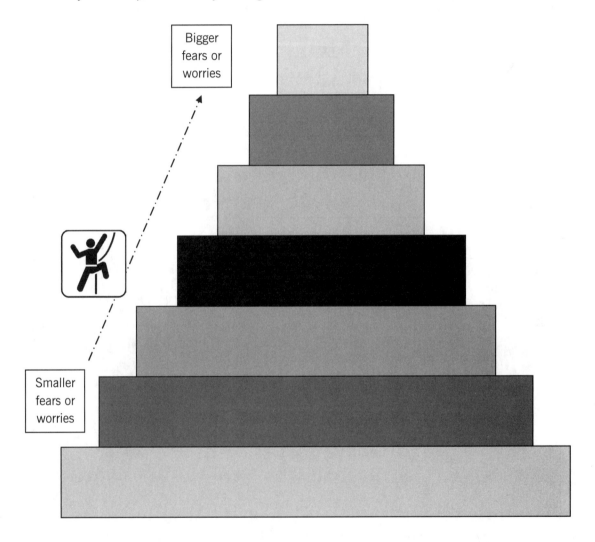

APPENDIX 4.5

SUDS Rating Scale

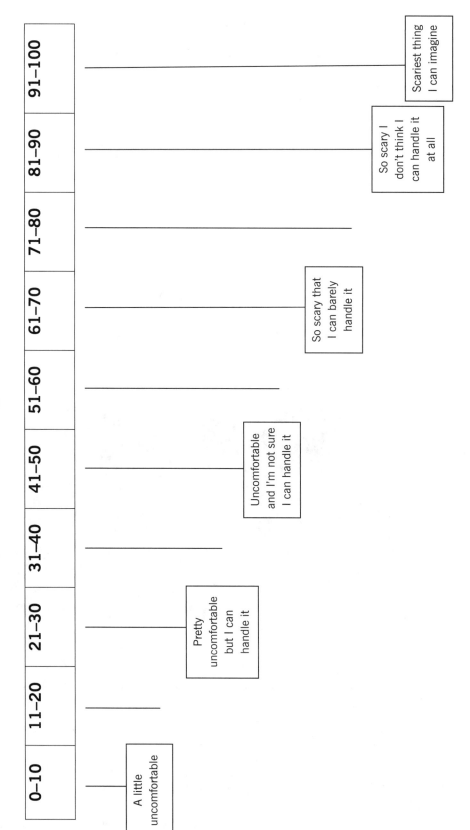

0–10	11–20	21–30	31–40	41–50	51–60	61–70	71–80	81–90	91–100

A little uncomfortable

Pretty uncomfortable but I can handle it

Uncomfortable and I'm not sure I can handle it

So scary that I can barely handle it

So scary I don't think I can handle it at all

Scariest thing I can imagine

Progressive Muscle Relaxation Exercise

Close your eyes and take a deep, deep breath . . . all the way down deep into your belly . . . Hold the breath for a second and then exhale . . . good . . . Now repeat this breathing . . . take another deep, deep breath, visualizing the air coming in through the soles of your feet and spreading upward, upward, upward, all the way to tip top of your head, collecting all the tension, the stress. Imagine this leaving your body as you exhale this breath. Now I would like you to focus on your body and how your body is feeling right now. Pay attention to how you feel . . . is your body heavy, is it light, is it tense, is it relaxed, do you feel calm, do you feel anxious? Go into your body and see how your body is feeling right now.

Now I'd like you to pay attention to your right hand . . . clench your right fist, making it tighter and tighter, tighter and tighter, good, hold it, hold it, hold it, and now relax . . . notice the contrast between a tight muscle and a loose one. Notice the pleasant sensation as the muscle relaxes.

Now I'd like you to pay attention to your left hand . . . clench your left fist, making it tighter and tighter, tighter and tighter, good, hold it, hold it, hold it, and now relax . . . notice the contrast . . . the contrast between a tight muscle and a loose one.

You are feeling more and more relaxed, deeply relaxed, calm, secure, stress free, and relaxed.

Now focus on your elbows and tense your biceps. Tense them as much as you can and notice the feelings of tightness . . . hold it, hold it, and now relax and straighten out your arms . . . let the relaxation flow all the way down your arms.

You are feeling more and more relaxed, deeply relaxed, calm, secure, stress free, and relaxed.

Now focus on your head and wrinkle your forehead as tight as you can . . . hold it, hold it, hold it, and now relax . . . smooth it out . . . let yourself imagine that your entire forehead is smooth, relaxed, smooth and relaxed.

Now clench your jaw, bite hard and notice the tension in your jaw . . . hold it, good, now relax. Really appreciate and feel the contrast between tension and relaxation in your jaw right now.

Now shrug your shoulders all the way up to the sky. Keep the tension as you hunch your head down between your shoulders, good, hold it, hold it. Now relax and feel the relaxation spreading through your neck, throat, and shoulders. Enjoy how loose and easy your neck now feels as it is balanced on your relaxed shoulders.

Now concentrate on your back. Arch it slightly, making sure not to strain. Focus on the tension in your lower back. Feel this tension and then relax. Focus on letting go of all the tension in the muscles of your lower back and abdomen.

You are feeling more and more relaxed, deeply relaxed, calm, secure, stress free, and relaxed.

Now curl your toes downward, making your calves tense. Study the tension and hold it, hold it, hold it, and now relax and enjoy the feelings of relaxation in your calves.

Now bend your toes toward your face, creating tension in your shins. Relax, enjoying the feeling of heaviness and peace that spreads everywhere in your legs.

Feel the heaviness in your entire body now. Enjoy it. Feel yourself heavier and heavier, heavier and heavier, more and more deeply relaxed. You feel calm, secure, relaxed, so deeply, deeply relaxed.

Based on a script by Tobin R. Lovell, PsyD, Georgia Southern University Counseling and Career Development Center. Retrieved April 17, 2010, from *www.allaboutdepression.com/relax/pmr/pmrscript.html*.

Breathing Exercise

After you get comfortable sitting where you are, we'll begin this exercise by taking several nice, long, deep breaths. Gently pull the air in, let it fill your lungs fully . . . then smoothly let it all out. Do this a few times as you let yourself get more relaxed sitting where you are. Breathe in fully let the air expand your lungs . . . then let the air flow easily back out again. While you are taking a few more deep breaths, notice if you are holding any tension in the muscles in your body. You might mentally scan your body, starting with your head. Notice your forehead, your cheeks, your jaw. Are you holding any tension in these areas? If so, just gently let all that tension melt away. Next, take notice of your neck, your shoulders, and upper back. If you are holding any tension here, again, just let all that tension go. Continue to mentally scan your body moving down to your arms and hands, your abdomen, and then your legs and feet. Gently let any tension in these areas just melt away. You might find that some tension creeps back into these muscle groups; that's okay. Just let it all go again with every out breath. Each time you breath out, let more and more tension leave your body. For a few more moments, bring your attention to your breathing . . . in and out. And, with every out-breath, let more and more tension melt away from your body.

As you are letting yourself become more relaxed sitting where you are, bring your attention to your breathing and begin to really notice how it feels. As you inhale, notice the cool air smoothly coming in through your nose or mouth, how it feels as it passes through your windpipe, gently filling your lungs. Notice the pause between the moment your lungs have fully filled with air, and the moment just before you exhale. Then notice how good it feels to let your full lungs collapse and how the warm air easily passes back through your windpipe and out through your nose or mouth. Likewise, notice that brief pause between the moment you fully exhale, and just before you inhale again. Bring your attention to your breathing . . . in and out . . . in and out. Notice the cool air coming in . . . filling your lungs . . . and the warm, soothing air flowing back out. With every out-breath, let more and more tension melt away. Noticing your breathing . . . in and out . . . in and out. If your mind wanders, that's OK, just gently bring your attention back to your breathing . . . in and out. Cool air coming in . . . filling your lungs . . . and the warm air gently flowing back out . . . in and out . . . in and out.

As you attend to your breathing, you might also begin to say a soothing word to yourself for the in-breath, and also for the out-breath. As you breath in, you might say to yourself, "peace." As you breath out, you might say, "release." On the in-breath "peace," and on the out-breath "release." Peace . . . release . . . peace . . . release. Bring your attention to your breathing . . . in and out. Peace . . . release . . . peace . . . release. If your mind wanders, that's OK, just gently bring your attention back to your breathing . . . in and out . . . in and out . . . in and out. With every out-breath, let more and more tension leave your body. Notice the cool air coming in . . . filling your lungs . . . and the warm, soothing air going back out. Bring your attention to your breathing . . . in and out . . . in and out . . . in and out. Continue this attention to your breathing for as long as you feel comfortable. And, when you feel ready, you can gently bring your attention back to the room while still letting yourself feel nice and comfortable and relaxed sitting where you are . . . noticing your breathing . . . in and out . . . in and out . . . in and out.

Based on a script by Prentiss Price, PhD, Georgia Southern University Counseling and Career Development Center. Retrieved April 17, 2010, *www.allaboutdepression.com/relax/deep2/deep2script.html*.

References

Albano, A. M., & Kendall, P. C. (2002). Cognitive behavioral therapy for children and adolescents with anxiety disorders: Clinical research advances. *International Review of Psychiatry, 14,* 129–134.

Baer, D., Wolf, M., & Risley, R. (1968). Some current dimensions of applied behavior analysis. *Journal of Applied Behavior Analysis, 1,* 91–97.

Baer, D., Wolf, M., & Risley, R. (1987). Some still-current dimensions of applied behavior analysis. *Journal of Applied Behavior Analysis, 20,* 313–327.

Barkley, R. (2000). *Taking charge of ADHD: The complete, authoritative guide for parents* (rev. ed.) New York: Guilford Press.

Beck, A. T. (1964). Thinking and depression: II. Theory and therapy. *Archives of General Psychiatry, 10,* 561–571.

Beck, A. T. (1976). *Cognitive therapy and the emotional disorders.* New York: International Universities Press.

Beck, A. T. (2005). The current state of cognitive therapy: A 40-year retrospective. *Archives of General Psychiatry, 62,* 953–959.

Beck, A. T., Emery, G., & Greenberg, R. L. (1990). *Anxiety disorders and phobias: A cognitive perspective.* New York: Basic Books.

Beck, A. T., Rush, A. J., Shaw, B. F., & Emory, G. (1979). *Cognitive therapy of depression.* John Wiley & Sons.

Beck, A. T., Wright, F. D., Newman, C. F., & Liese, B. S. (1993). *Cogntive therapy of substance abuse.* New York: Guilford Press.

Beck, J. S. (1995). *Cognitive therapy: Basics and beyond.* New York: Guilford Press.

Beidas, R. S., & Kendall, P. C. (2010). Training therapists in evidence-based practice: A critical review of studies from a systems-contextual perspective. *Clinical Psychology: Science and Practice, 17,* 1–30.

Bennett, H., & Wells, A. (2010). Metacognition, memory disorganization, and rumination in post-traumatic stress symptoms. *Journal of Anxiety Disorders, 24,* 318–325.

Benson, H. (1975). *The relaxation response.* New York: Avon.

Bernstein, G. A., Layne, A. E., Egan, E. A. & Tennison, D. M. (2005). School-based interventions for anxious children. *Journal of the American Academy of Child and Adolescent Psychiatry, 44,* 1118–1127.

Bloomquist, M. L., August, G. J., & Ostrander, R. (1991). Effects of a school-based cognitive-behavioral intervention for ADHD children. *Journal of Abnormal Child Psychology, 19,* 591–605.

Braswell, L., & Bloomquist, M. L. (1991). *Cognitive-behavioral therapy with ADHD children: Child, family, and school interventions.* New York: Guilford Press.

Burns, D. D. (1980). *Feeling good: The new mood therapy.* New York: Signet.

Butler, A. C., Chapman, J. E., Forman, E. M., & Beck, A. T. (2006). The empirical status of cognitive-behavioral therapy: A review of meta-analyses. *Clinical Psychology Review, 26*(1), 17–31.

Centers for Disease Control and Prevention, National Center for Injury Prevention and Control. (2006). Web-based Injury Statistics Query and Reporting System (WISQARS): *www.cdc.gov/ncipc/wisqars.*

Chambless, D. L., & Ollendick, T. H. (2001). Empirically supported psychological interventions: Controversies and evidence. *Annual Review of Psychology, 52,* 685–716.

Cisler, J. M., & Koster, E. H. W. (2010). Mechanisms of attentional biases towards threat in anxiety disorders: An integrative review. *Clinical Psychology Review, 30,* 203–216.

Clarke, G., Lewinsohn, P., & Hops, H. (1990). *Instructor's manual for the Adolescent Coping with Depression Course.* Eugene, OR: Castalia Press.

Clerkin, E. M., & Teachman, B. A. (2010). Training implicit social anxiety associations: An experimental intervention. *Journal of Anxiety Disorders, 24,* 300–308.

Coffman, S. J., Martell, C. R., Dimidjian, S., Gallop, R., & Hollon, S. D. (2007). Extreme nonresponse in cognitive therapy: Can behavioral activation succeed where cognitive therapy fails? *Journal of Consulting and Clinical Psychology, 75,* 531–541.

Cohen, J. A., Deblinger, E., Mannarino, A. P., & Steer, R. (2004). A multi-site randomized controlled trial for children with sexual abuse-related PTSD. *Journal of the American Academy of Child and Adolescent Psychiatry 43*(4), 393–402.

Cottraux, J., Note, I., Albuisson, E., Yao, S. N., Note, B., Mollard, E., et al. (2000). Cognitive behavior therapy versus supportive therapy in social phobia: A randomized controlled trial. *Psychotherapy and Psychosomatics, 69,* 137–146.

Cromer, L. D., & Smyth, J. M. (2010). Making meaning of trauma: Trauma exposure doesn't tell the whole story. *Journal of Contemporary Psychotherapy, 4*(0), 65–72.

Crone, D. A., & Horner, R. H. (2003). *Building positive behavior support systems in schools.* New York: Guilford Press.

Davidson, J. R. T., Foa, E. B., Huppert, J. D., Keefe, F., Franklin, M., Compton, J., et al. (2004). Fluoxetine, comprehensive cognitive behavioral therapy, and placebo in generalized social phobia. *Archives of General Psychiatry, 61,* 1005–1013.

Deblinger E., Stauffer L. B., & Steer R. A. (2001). Comparative efficacies of supportive and cognitive behavioral group therapies for young children who have been sexually abused and their non-offending mothers. *Child Maltreatment, 6,* 332–343.

DeRubeis, R. J. & Feeley, M. (1990). Determinants of change in cognitive therapy for depression. *Cognitive Therapy and Research, 14,* 469–482.

Edelman, R. E., & Chambless, D. L. (1995). Adherence during sessions and homework in cognitive behavioral group treatment of social phobia. *Behaviour Research and Therapy, 33,* 573–577.

Foa, E. B., Dancu, C. V., Hembree, E. A., Jaycox, L. H., Meadows, E. A., & Street, G. P. (1999). A comparison of exposure therapy, stress inoculation training, and their combination for reducing posttraumatic stress disorder in female assault victims. *Journal of Consulting and Clinical Psychology, 67,* 194–200.

Foa, E. B., Hembree, E. A., Cahill, S. P., Rauch, S. A. M., Riggs, D. S., Feeny, N. C., et al. (2005). Randomized trial of prolonged exposure for posttraumatic stress disorder with and without cognitive restructuring: Outcome at academic and community clinics. *Journal of Consulting and Clinical Psychology, 73,* 953–964.

Foa, E. B., Rothbaum, B. O., Riggs, D., & Murdock, T. (1991). Treatment of post-traumatic stress disorder in rape victims: A comparison between cognitive-behavioral procedures and counseling. *Journal of Consulting and Clinical Psychology, 59,* 715–723.

Foa, E. B., Steketee, G., Grayson, J. B., Turner, R. M., & Latimer, P. (1984). Deliberate exposure and blocking of obsessive–compulsive rituals: Immediate and long-term effects. *Behavior Therapy, 15,* 450–472.

Foa, E. B., Steketee, G. S., & Milby, J. B. (1980). Differential effects of exposure and response prevention in obsessive–compulsive washers. *Journal of Consulting and Clinical Psychology, 48,* 71–79.

Foa, E. B., Steketee, G., Turner, R. M., & Fischer, S. C. (1980). Effects of imaginal exposure to feared disasters in obsessive–compulsive checkers. *Behaviour Research and Therapy, 18,* 449–455.

Franklin, M. E., Abramowitz, J. S., Kozak, M. J., Levitt, J. T., & Foa, E. B. (2000). Effectiveness of exposure and ritual prevention for obsessive–compulsive disorder: Randomized compared with nonrandomized samples. *Journal of Consulting and Clinical Psychology, 68,* 594–602.

Gimpel Peacock, G., & Collett, B. R. (2010). *Collaborative home/school interventions: Evidence-based solutions for emotional, behavioral, and academic problems.* New York: Guilford Press.

Gotestam, K. G., & Hokstad, A. (2002). One session treatment of spider phobia in a group setting with rotating active exposure. *European Journal of Psychiatry, 16,* 129–134.

Gotlib, I. H., & Joormann, J. (2010). Cognition and depression: Current status and future directions. *Annual Review of Clinical Psychology, 6,* 285–312.

Granholm, E., McQuaid, J. R., Auslander, L., & McClure, F. S. (2004). Group cognitive behavioral social skills training for outpatients with chronic schizophrenia. *Journal of Cognitive Therapy: An International Quarterly, 18,* 265–279.

Granholm, E., McQuaid, J. R., McClure, F. S., Auslander, L. A., Perivoliotis, D., Pedrelli, P., Patterson, T., & Jeste, D. V. (2005). A randomized controlled trial of cognitive behavioral social skills training for middle aged and older outpatients with chronic schizophrenia. *American Journal of Psychiatry, 162,* 520–529.

Grossman, P. B., & Hughes, J. N. (1992). Self-control interventions with internalizing disorders: A review and analysis. *School Psychology Review, 21*(2), 229–245.

Hayes, S. C., Follette, V. M., & Linehan, M. M. (2004). *Mindfulness and acceptance: Expanding the cognitive behavioral tradition.* New York: Guilford Press.

Heimberg, R. G., Dodge, C. S., Hope, D. A., Kennedy, C. R., Zollo, L. J., & Becker, R. E. (2000). Cognitive behavioral group treatment for social phobia: Comparison with a credible placebo control. *Cognitive Therapy and Research, 14,* 1–23.

Jacobson, E. (1974). *Progressive relaxation.* Chicago: University of Chicago Press, Midway Reprint.

Kendall, P. C., Hudson, J., Gosch, E., Flannery-Schroeder, E., & Suveg, C. (2008). Cognitive-behavioral therapy for anxiety disordered youth: A randomized clinical trial evaluating child and family modalities. *Journal of Consulting and Clinical Psychology, 76,* 282–297.

Kendall, P. C., Hudson, J. L., Choudhury, M., Webb, A., & Pimentel, S. (2005). Cognitive-behavioral treatment for childhood anxiety disorders. In E. D. Hibbs & P. S. Jensen (Eds.), *Psychosocial treatments for child and adolescent disorders: Empirically based strategies for clinical practice* (2nd ed., pp. 47–73). Washington, DC: American Psychological Association.

Ladouceur, R., Dugas, M. J., Freeston, M. H., Léger, E., Gagnon, F., & Thibodeau, N. (2000). Efficacy of cognitive-behavioral treatment of generalized anxiety disorder: Evaluation in a controlled clinical trial. *Journal of Consulting and Clinical Psychology, 68,* 957–964.

Landon, T. M., & Barlow, D. H. (2004). Cognitive-behavioral treatment for panic disorder: Current status. *Journal of Psychiatric Practice, 10,* 211–226.

Lee, N. K., Pohlman, S., Baker, A., Ferris, J., & Kay-Lambkin, F. (2010). It's the thought that counts: Craving metacognitions and their role in abstinence from methamphetamine use. *Journal of Substance Abuse Treatment, 38,* 245–250.

Leung, A. W., & Heimberg, R. G. (1996). Homework compliance, perceptions of control and outcome in cognitive behavioral treatment for social phobia. *Behaviour Research and Therapy, 34,* 423–432.

March, J. S. (1995). Cognitive-behavioral psychotherapy for children and adolescents with OCD: A review and recommendations for treatment. *Journal of the American Academy of Child and Adolescent Psychiatry. 34*(1), 7–18.

Mawson, A., Cohen, K., & Berry, K. (2010). Reviewing evidence for the cognitive model of auditory hallucinations: The relationship between cognitive voice appraisals and distress during psychosis. *Clinical Psychology Review, 30,* 248–258.

Moats, L. C., & Hall, S. L. (1999). *Straight talk about reading: How parents can make a difference during the early years.* New York: Contemporary Books.

Moss, D., McGrady, A., Davies, T. C., & Wickramasekera, I. (2003). *Handbook of mind–body medicine for primary care.* Thousand Oaks, CA: Sage.

Muhlberger, A., Wiedemann, G. C., & Pauli, P. (2003). Efficacy of a one-session virtual reality exposure treatment for fear of flying. *Psychotherapy Research, 13,* 323–336.

Muñoz, R. F., Ippen, C. G., Rao, S., Le, H.-N., & Dwyer, E. V. (2000). *Manual for group cognitive-behavioral therapy of major depression.* San Francisco: University of California. Available at *medschool. ucsf. edu/latino/manuals. aspx.*

Neimeyer, R. A., & Feixas, G. (1990). The role of homework and skill acquisition in the outcome of group cognitive therapy for depression. *Behavior Therapy,21,* 281–292.

O'Kearney, R. T., Anstey, K. J., & von Sanden, C. (2006). Behavioural and cognitive behavioura therapy for obsessive compulsive disorder in children and adolescents (Review). *Cochrane Database of Systematic Reviews, 4.*

O'Neill, R. E., Horner, R. H., Alpine, R. W., Sprague, J. R., Storey, K., & Newton, J. S. (1997). *Functional assessment and program development for problem behavior* (2nd Ed.). Pacific Grove, CA: Cole Publishing Company.

Öst, L. G., Alm, T., Brandberg, M., & Breitholtz, E. (2001). One vs. five sessions of exposure and five sessions of cognitive therapy in the treatment of claustrophobia. *Behaviour Research and Therapy, 39*(2), 167–183.

Persons, J. B., & Burns, D. D. (1985). Mechanisms of action of cognitive therapy: The relative contributions of technical and interpersonal interventions. *Cognitive Therapy and Research, 9,* 539–551.

Rees, C. S., McEvoy, P., & Nathan, P. R. (2005). Relationship between homework completion and outcome in cognitive behaviour therapy. *Cognitive Behaviour Therapy, 34*(4), 242–247.

Reinecke, M. A., Ryan, N. E., & DuBois, D. L. (1998). Cognitive-behavioral therapy of depression and depressive symptoms during adolescence: A review and meta-analysis. *Journal of the American Academy of Child and Adolescent Psychiatry,37*(1), 26–34.

Resick, P. A., Nishith, P., Weaver, T. L., Astin, M. C., & Feuer, C. A. (2002). A comparison of cognitive-processing therapy with prolonged exposure and a waiting condition for the treatment of chronic posttraumatic stress disorder in female rape victims. *Journal of Consulting and Clinical Psychology, 70*, 867–879.

Romens, S. E., Abramson L. Y., & Alloy, A. B. (2009). High and low cognitive risk for depression: Stability from late adolescence to early adulthood. *Cognitive Therapy and Research, 33*, 480–498.

Ruffolo, M. C., & Fischer, D. (2009). Using an evidence-based CBT group intervention model for adolescents with depressive symptoms: Lessons learned from a school-based adaptation. *Child and Family Social Work, 14*, 189–197.

Segal, Z. V., Gemar, M., & Williams, S. (1999). Differential cognitive response to a mood challenge following successful cognitive therapy or pharmacotherapy for unipolar depression. *Journal of Abnormal Psychology, 108*, 3–10.

Segal, Z. V., Kennedy, S., Gemar, M., Hood, K., Pedersen, R., & Buis, T. (2006). Cognitive reactivity to sad mood provocation and the prediction of depressive relapse. *Archives of General Psychiatry, 63*, 749–755.

Selekman, M. D. (1993). *Pathways to change: Brief therapy solutions with difficult adolescents*. New York: Guilford Press.

Shirk, S. R., Kaplinski, H., & Gudmundsen, G. (2009). School-based cognitive-behavioral therapy for adolescent depression: A benchmarking study. *Journal of Emotional and Behavioral Disorders, 17*, 106–117.

Smith, D. C., Larson, J., & Nuckles, D. R. (2006). A critical analysis of school-based anger management programs for youth. In S. R. Jimerson & M. Furlong (Eds.), *Handbook of school violence and school safety: From research to practice* (pp. 365–382). Mahwah, NJ: Erlbaum.

Stanford, E. J., Goetz, R. R., & Bloom, J. D. (1994). The no harm contract in the emergency assessment of suicidal risk. *Journal of Clinical Psychiatry,55*, 344–348.

Stanley, B., Brown, G., Brent, D. A., Wells, K., Poling, K., Curry, J., et al. (2009). Cognitive-behavioral therapy for suicide prevention (CBT-SP): Treatment model, feasibility, and acceptability. *Journal of the American Academy of Child and Adolescent Psychiatry, 48*, 1005–1013.

Stirman, S. W., Bhar, S. S., Spokas, M., Brown, G. K., Creed, T. A., Perivoliotis, D., et al. (2010). Training and consultation in evidence-based psychosocial treatments in public mental health settings: The ACCESS model. *Professional Psychology: Research and Practice, 41*, 48–56.

Syzdek, M. R., Addis, M. E., & Martell, C. R. (2010). Working with emotion and emotion regulation in behavioral activation treatment for depressed mood. In A. M. Kring, & D. M. Sloan (Eds.), *Emotion regulation and psychopathology: A transdiagnostic approach to etiology and treatment* (pp. 405–426). New York: Guilford Press.

Treatment for Adolescents with Depression Study (TADS) Team. (2004). Fluoxetine, cognitive-behavioral therapy, and their combination for adolescents with depression: Treatment for adolescents with depression study (TADS) randomized controlled trial. *Journal of the American Medical Association, 292*, 807–820.

Van Oppen, P., de Haan, E., Van Balkom, A. J. L. M., & Spinhoven, P. (1995). Cognitive therapy and exposure in vivo in the treatment of obsessive compulsive disorder. *Behaviour Research and Therapy, 33*, 379–390.

Wenzel, A., Brown, G. K., & Beck, A. T. (2009). *Cognitive therapy for suicidal patients: Scientific and clinical applications*. Washington, DC: American Psychological Association.

Willumsen, T., Vassend, O., & Hoffart, A. (2001). A comparison of cognitive therapy, applied relaxation, and nitrous oxide sedation in the treatment of dental fear. *Acta Odontologica Scandinavica, 59,* 290–296.

Wolpe, J. (1969). *The practice of behavior therapy*. New York: Pergamon Press.

Index